Humans in Nature

Humans in Nature

The World As We Find It and the World As We Create It

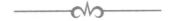

Gregory E. Kaebnick

OXFORD
UNIVERSITY PRESS

OXFORD
UNIVERSITY PRESS

Oxford University Press is a department of the University of Oxford.
It furthers the University's objective of excellence in research, scholarship,
and education by publishing worldwide.

Oxford   New York

Auckland   Cape Town   Dar es Salaam   Hong Kong   Karachi
Kuala Lumpur   Madrid   Melbourne   Mexico City   Nairobi
New Delhi   Shanghai   Taipei   Toronto

With offices in

Argentina   Austria   Brazil   Chile   Czech Republic   France   Greece
Guatemala   Hungary   Italy   Japan   Poland   Portugal   Singapore
South Korea   Switzerland   Thailand   Turkey   Ukraine   Vietnam

Oxford is a registered trademark of Oxford University Press
in the UK and certain other countries.

Published in the United States of America by
Oxford University Press
198 Madison Avenue, New York, NY 10016

Library of Congress Cataloging–in–Publication Data
Kaebnick, Gregory E.
Humans in nature: the world as we find it and the world as
we create it / Gregory E. Kaebnick.
pages cm
Includes bibliographical references.
ISBN 978–0–19–934721–6 (hardcover : alk. paper)
1. Philosophy of nature.   2. Nature—Effect of human beings on.   I. Title.
BD581.K34 2013
113—dc23
2013022729

1 3 5 7 9 8 6 4 2

To Rebecca, who wants to live richly within the natural bounds of life; to Hannah, who wants to live forever (and have wings); and to Gwen, who wants all good things for our children.

CONTENTS

PREFACE

Technology—the modification of nature for the further modification of nature—is celebrated as one of the marks of human nature. Yet many people are also increasingly concerned about the depth and extent to which our technological prowess now allows humans to modify nature, human and otherwise: they are concerned, for example, about the human-caused extinction of plants and animals, about the introduction of genetically engineered crops and livestock, and about the biotechnological enhancement of human beings. Similar concerns have been expressed about the field of synthetic biology, which aims to bring engineering to biology and make possible the construction of organisms designed to serve human ends.

All of these concerns are about the desirability of altering natural states of affairs—human nature, animal and plant nature, and nature in the environment around us. They are not just fears that the alterations will turn out to be bad for human welfare; to some extent, they are misgivings about the very idea of altering natural states of affairs, regardless of the possible consequences for anyone's welfare. Wiping out the nautilus to make baubles from its shells may well be a rational thing to do from the standpoint of human benefit, but many would still think it awful. Introducing a jellyfish gene into zebrafish to create the fluorescing Glofish, a highlight for any aquarium, is probably unexceptionable from the standpoint of human benefit, and yet it makes some people a bit queasy. The prospect of significantly altering human beings, if the alterations are not aimed at treating disease, is also an unattractive prospect to at least some ordinary human beings. In such cases, a natural state of affairs is held to be *intrinsically* morally significant: people care about that state morally and have an urge to preserve it, for its own sake, rather than because of some other valuable thing that it may be useful for attaining.

These widely and deeply felt intuitions about the destruction of naturally occurring spaces and species and about the use of biotechnologies to

change crops and livestock or to enhance human beings face several serious challenges. First, can we ever really identify a "natural" state of affairs?
The world as found and the world as created or altered can be hard to tease
apart. The few remaining patches of tallgrass prairie look to be natural, for
example, but they require extensive human management to stay that way,
and some of them are the result of "restoration" efforts that may seem to
be examples as clear as any of human intervention into nature. Even the
"original" prairies, those that white settlers found in their westward trek,
were managed: they had been maintained by deliberately set fires, and the
mix of species that European settlers found in them was quite different
from what it had been about 15,000 years earlier.

Second, why should we value nature? Can it make sense to say that we
value nature morally? The standard accounts of moral values in the Western
philosophical canon do not easily accommodate moral concerns about
human activity that drives species into extinction or might lead to fundamental changes in human nature. To many critics, objections to changing
nature demonstrate irrationality; morality calls precisely for changing the
world as we find it to make it better.

Third, even if we can come up with answers to the first two questions,
still, how should moral concerns about nature be taken up into public discourse and public policy making? Should they? Or should government
strive to be neutral on such matters? In the Western liberal tradition, the
range of acceptable government action is often thought to be restricted,
and individuals are given considerable latitude to live by their own values. If so, then however we settle the moral question, perhaps individuals
should be left to commune with nature or remake it as they please.

This book, which emerges from a series of projects that The Hastings
Center has conducted with funding from the National Endowment for
the Humanities, the Alfred P. Sloan Foundation, the National Institutes
of Health, the Rockefeller Foundation, and the United States Anti-Doping
Association, explores questions about the moral significance of "nature" or
"the natural" in two ways. The first four chapters isolate the philosophical
challenges and propose approaches to them that will make possible a careful, sympathetic, yet critical examination of specific concerns about the
ways humans alter nature. The second half works within this framework
to conduct a comparative analysis of some of those concerns. Each chapter
looks at how the concept of "nature" is deployed in a different social debate
and how the deployment fares. Four debates are examined in depth: arguments about preserving the environment (ecosystems, "wildernesses," and
endangered species, for example), about genetically altering livestock and
crops, about synthetic biology, and about human enhancement. In the

course of considering these debates, these chapters also provide an opportunity to further explore and elaborate the framework developed earlier. The chapters are intended both to complement each other and to work independently.

The rationale for setting these seemingly diverse problems alongside each other is that the comparisons might be illuminating. The literature on environmentalist concerns, for example, might suggest new ways of thinking about the human enhancement debate; concerns about human enhancement have seemed to founder on the difficulty of identifying a natural state of affairs or of explaining why it can have intrinsic value, and environmentalist philosophy provides resources that could help overcome those problems. On the other hand, comparisons across debates might in some cases allay a concern or show its limitations. The concerns that have been expressed about synthetic biology draw on but also contrast with concerns about human alteration of the environment, for example, and the contrast might lead to a reevaluation of the sense in which synthetic biology really changes the human relationship to nature. In short, both the commonalities and the differences across these topics need attention. The fact that there are linkages among the various debates about the human alteration of nature does not mean that they are all of a piece. At the end of the day, within these different debates, one may reach fundamentally different views about the moral ideal of preserving nature.

Conducting the study in a comparative fashion also addresses a gap of sorts in the literature—or really, the literatures. Much has been written about human enhancement, much about agricultural biotechnology, and much about the status of the environment, but, for the most part, these discussions have occurred in isolation from each other. Bioethicists mostly do not read journals that publish on agricultural ethics and environmental ethics, and scholars in environmental ethics mostly do not think of themselves as doing bioethics or agricultural ethics. As a result, their approaches to concerns about nature can easily seem ad hoc and disconnected.

For example, critiques of human biotechnology sometimes seek to show how moral values are tied to human nature: Leon Kass argues that human embodiment is connected to the concept of human dignity, whereas Jürgen Habermas, coming at the issue from a very different political perspective, argues that parents should not enhance their children because doing so would undermine the child's capacity for autonomy. Neither approach obviously lends itself to making sense of concerns about animal nature or the environment. Objections to agricultural biotechnology, on the other hand, sometimes rest on claims about the value of preserving "animal integrity" or "species integrity," which involve claims about species norms and holistic functioning. These views might be adapted to underwrite criticisms of human biotechnology, but they have no immediate relevance to debates about preserving the environment. Meanwhile, some environmental philosophers have considered whether ecosystems and trees may themselves have value, understanding value as a property that exists in the universe independently of human interests, and they have looked for metaphysical theories that would make sense of that conception of value. But how that kind of account would apply to human biotechnology is an open question.

These arguments should be in dialogue with each other. The problems are not quite as diverse as the disconnectedness of their treatment would suggest. On the face of it, the reservations many people have about agricultural and medical biotechnology and human overhaul of the environment appear to be analogs to some degree, given that they are all about the value of accepting natural states of affairs, of resisting the societal drive to reengineer all the world. If, at the end of the day, we reach fundamentally different conclusions on different topics, then there must be differences in how the concerns are developed, but, given the underlying base similarities among the concerns, it is well worth looking carefully for an account that recognizes the similarities.

There are many other social debates that invoke the concept of nature than those discussed here; claims about what is natural also appear in debates about sexual practices, gender roles, race relations, assisted reproduction, and parenting. Some of the discussion in this book has implications for these topics: debates about whether homosexuality is intrinsically undesirable (because unnatural) could draw on observations offered in Chapter 2 about moral argument and on some positions developed in Chapter 8 about how claims about human nature figure in morality, about the distinction between population norms and individual differences, and about the extent to which human beings are self-creating entities. But while these other debates should eventually be addressed in order to thoroughly examine the concept of nature, they are not front and center in this book. The debates taken up here—about environmental preservation, genetically modified organisms in agriculture, synthetic biology, and human enhancement—revolve around the contrast between preserving or altering one or another existing state of affairs. These other debates have more to do with whether states of affairs believed to be natural provide guidance for human relationships with each other. The idea of nature can still figure in these topics in complex ways; I have argued in another place, for example, that a biological relationship with one's children cannot be privileged above adoptive relationships on grounds that one is natural and the other merely social, but also that where there is a biological relationship, that fact can become a very meaningful part of that parent–child relationship. But a complete discussion of these other topics is not attempted here.

Also, for those topics that are taken up here, there are many other moral arguments to be weighed than are discussed here. The debate about environmental protection, for example, is moving beyond local concerns—preservation of particular wild spaces and species—toward planetary problems—prevention or correction of global warming, air pollution, and ocean acidification. Chapter 5 mentions such issues but does not address them in detail. These concerns are extremely urgent, but they can be handled by means of relatively traditional moral concepts, without invoking the idea that nature is intrinsically valuable. In fact, some environmentalists argue against the kinds of moral concerns addressed at length in Chapter 5 on grounds that they distract from the really serious, global environmental problems. Whether that is true, in my view, is a question of political strategy more than of morality.

The ultimate goal of the book is to mark out a middle way—to provide a way of thinking about the human relationship to nature that neither leaves all objections to altering nature standing nor wipes them all off the table as illegitimate. At least within academia, this middle way has been elusive. Scholarly debates have tended toward extreme polarization, with some scholars suggesting that concerns about altering nature are profoundly important whereas others argue that they are irrational, even incoherent. The overarching theme in this book is that they can be legitimate and serious, but also that they are complex, contestable, and limited: they are not a kind of moral trump card, capable of closing down a debate. Nor do they work equally well in every debate in which they are articulated. Nor does every way of articulating them—for there are several—work equally well. But precisely by recognizing these difficulties, we can make sense of them.

ACKNOWLEDGMENTS

The development of these ideas must be credited primarily to the rich conversations I have had at The Hastings Center with all of the scholars and visitors there, but especially with Erik Parens, Thomas Murray, Daniel Callahan, Bruce Jennings, and Strachan Donnelley. I am also deeply indebted to the participants of a number of research projects in which I have been involved at Hastings, and especially to the participants of "The Ideal of Nature: Appeals to Nature in Debates about Biotechnology and the Environment," funded by the National Endowment for the Humanities, "Ethical Issues in Synthetic Biology," funded by the Alfred P. Sloan Foundation, and "The Ethical Issues of Synthetic Biology: An Examination of Four Cases," also funded by Sloan. Participants who were particularly helpful, reading chapters and weeding out mistakes, are Mark Bedau, Rob Carlson, Jon Mandle, and Peter Murray. Strachan and Bruce were also kind enough to invite me into some fascinating and very helpful discussions at the Center for Humans and Nature, after they moved there from Hastings. And, although it is now some years since I finished my doctoral studies, I still owe an ongoing debt to my advisor at the University of Minnesota, Eugene Mason.

I have tested out some of the ideas in this book by attempting to articulate them in various formats—to audiences at the University of Minnesota, Yale University, the University of California at Berkeley, the University of Oklahoma, Purdue University, the University of Tokyo, and Freiburg University, and in several previously published papers. Chapter 2 builds on "Reasons of the Heart: Emotions, Rationality, and the 'Wisdom of Repugnance,'" published in the *Hastings Center Report* in 2008 (volume 38, number 4); Chapter 6 incorporates elements from "Putting Concerns About Nature in Context: The Case of Agricultural Biotechnology," published in *Perspectives in Biology and Medicine*; Chapter 7 is based closely on "Engineered Microbes in Industry and

Science: A New Human Relationship to Nature?," published in *Synthetic Biology and Morality: Artificial Life and the Bounds of Nature* (MIT Press, 2013); and Chapter 8 draws on "Human Nature Without Theory," in *The Ideal of Nature: Debates About Biotechnology and the Environment* (Johns Hopkins University Press, 2011).

CHAPTER 1

The Nature of "Nature"

What to Ask of a Concept

It is often extremely difficult to identify a "natural" state of affairs. Is the tallgrass prairie "natural," or does the fact that human beings maintained it by regularly setting fires establish that an entire ecosystem we associate with the American Midwest was actually a kind of human artifact? What about cows or corn, bred respectively from the now-extinct European aurochs and from one or another species of the Mexican grass known as *teosinte*? Is an uncommonly muscular human body "natural" if it is achieved through the use of steroids and human growth hormone? How does it compare to a similar body sculpted only by means of careful food choices and a rigorous weight-lifting regimen? Or what if it were achieved instead by modifying the person's genes?

Such questions have led many commentators to dismiss the concept of nature as unsustainable. Nonetheless, the concept is still often taken for granted in ordinary conversation. Kate Soper leads off her complex and extended exploration of what "nature" means by emphasizing just this point:

> Its complexity is concealed by the ease and regularity with which we put it to
> use in a wide variety of contexts. It is at once both very familiar and extremely
> elusive: an idea we employ with such ease and regularity that it seems as if we
> ourselves are privileged with some "natural" access to its intelligibility; but also

an idea which most of us know, in some sense, to be so various and comprehensive in its use as to defy our powers of definition.[1]

The difficulty of understanding how to think about the concept of nature is possibly the most fundamental problem in getting clear on whether leaving nature alone can ever be morally desirable. It is certainly the *threshold* problem; we must consider it before there is any point in turning to some of the further problems that arise.

There are actually two parts to the problem. First is a problem of finding a suitable definition of "nature." The concept can seem too multifarious and vague, an assortment of possible meanings that are individually unworkable and collectively a useless jumble. "Nature" can refer to the world prior to or independent of human meddling, or to a state of human life prior to the complications of civilization, or to the realm of things suitable for scientific investigation, or to the typical make-up of kinds of things (the *nature* of rocks, or cows, or humans), or to the unique make-up of particular things (as in, "it's in his nature to do that"). It can refer to what's growing in the garden or to what the gardener tries to keep out of the garden or to the forces that the gardener is sometimes grumblingly dependent on. "Natural" may mean "in accordance with physical or biological regularities," or "unaltered," or "unadorned and honest,"[2] or "typical and acceptable" (as opposed to perverse). It may mean "predictable," as in, "Naturally, the plumber didn't show up on time…"; or something akin to "rational" or "sensible," as in "The natural conclusion is that…"; or "unaffected" or "at ease," as in "Try to look natural…."

The second problem is that the understanding of "nature" might be a cultural construction—a historical development that could have gone differently and that happened only recently. If so, can the concept be legitimate? More than once when I have mentioned to somebody my interest in moral attitudes about the human relationship to nature, that person has set the whole inquiry aside with a wave of the hand: "Oh, 'nature.' That's a nineteenth-century invention, you know."

The two problems are distinguishable. The first has to do with coherence and the second with justification: the first charges that "nature" admits no useful definition and the second that particular definitions are not grounded in the way they should be to be morally useful. The problems are related, though. Both charge that the distinctions typically drawn between "natural" and "not natural" do not describe the world appropriately—that they do not group things together coherently (the first problem), perhaps because they are not guided by the world as it really is (the second problem). Thus, both suggest the ultimate indefensibility of the distinction between "natural" and "not natural."

ARE HUMANS COMPATIBLE WITH NATURE?

The debate about how to define nature goes back a ways. The definitive critique was set out by John Stuart Mill, in an eloquent and indignant essay called simply "On Nature." Mill argued that "nature" usually means one of two things: "In one sense, it means all the powers existing in either the outer or the inner world and everything which takes place by means of those powers. In another sense it means, not everything which happens, but only what takes place without the agency, or without the voluntary and intentional agency of man."[3] Neither of the meanings, however, supports any recommendations for action: if "nature" means everything that conforms to the laws of physics, then everything is natural, including whatever humans may do to the world around them. If "natural" refers only to that which is free of human interference, then *nothing* we do is natural. Either way, the concept tells us nothing about what we do to nature and cannot be used to make any distinctions about good, acceptable, undesirable, or outright wrong kinds of things that we can do to nature.

The first thing to note is that the concept of nature can have different uses in moral argument and that Mill is criticizing a particularly ambitious way of using it. Mill's objection is to the idea that nature provides *moral guidance*: "When it is asserted or implied that nature, or the laws of nature, should be conformed to, is the nature which is meant nature in the first sense of the term, meaning all which is...?"[4] This makes no sense, Mill explains: "Man necessarily obeys the laws of nature, or, in other words, the properties of things, but does not necessarily *guide* himself by them."[5] And, if we take "nature" in the second sense, as that which takes place without human intervention, then taking our cue from nature would simply be wrong. "In sober truth, nearly all the things which men are hanged or imprisoned for doing to one another are nature's everyday performances."[6] If we are trying to determine how people should treat each other, then, we do particularly poorly to turn to nature for ideas. As Bonnie Steinbock puts the point in an examination of Mill's critique, "nature is not the source of substantive moral rules."[7]

Another, much more modest way in which the concept of "nature" can enter into morality, however, is that it could be a *subject* of moral guidance; as Steinbock also notes, it can and should have value. Here, nature is not a guide to morality, but a topic within morality. The issue is the value of nature, not obedience to nature. Mill himself writes about the value of nature:

Nor is there much satisfaction in contemplating the world with nothing left to the spontaneous activity of Nature; with every rood of land brought into cultivation which is capable of producing food for human beings; every flowering waste or nature pasture ploughed up, all quadrupeds or birds which are not domesticated for man's use exterminated as his rivals for food, every hedgerow or superfluous tree rooted out, and scarcely a place left where a wild shrub or flower could grow without being eradicated in the name of improved agriculture.[8]

The question still arises, however: how can we individuate a "natural state of affairs" that we might want to leave alone? Mill's critique must still be answered in some way, for it implies that there is no way of saying which human actions would leave nature alone. This point has been picked up by various modern commentators. In bioethics, it was picked up prominently by the President's Commission for the Study of Ethical Problems in Medicine and Biomedical and Behavioral Research, which issued a handful of very influential reports in the early 1980s on various bioethical topics. In *Splicing Life: A Report on the Social and Ethical Issues of Genetic Engineering with Human Beings*, the commission offered an ultimately dismissive analysis of the objection that genetic engineering amounted to "playing God." The analysis echoed Mill:

> [I]n one sense *all* human activity that produces changes that otherwise would not have occurred interferes with nature. Medical activities as routine as the prescription of eyeglasses for myopia or replacement of a damaged heart are in this sense "unnatural." In another sense, human activity cannot interfere with nature—in the sense of contravening it—since all human activities, including gene splicing, proceed according to the scientific laws that describe natural processes.[9]

In discussions of agricultural biotechnology, too, the point is commonly made that everything about agriculture, for thousands of years, has been an instance of human interference into the nature of organisms and environment and is therefore all equally outside the pale of nature. Or, turning to a version of Mill's first claim about nature, it is all equally natural: even the fanciest sorts of biotechnological interventions, such as splicing genes from one organism into another, merely mimic things that already go on in nature. (Microorganisms very readily transfer genes across species lines.[10])

The problem of defining "nature" has also seemed insuperable to some environmental philosophers. Steven Vogel has argued, for example, that the concept of nature can provide no ground for guidance as to how humans should behave toward nature if "nature" has only the two meanings Mill identifies. With neither meaning "can we make much sense out of claims, for instance, that certain human practices or products are more 'natural' than others: we either are already guaranteed to be fully natural or else we are guaranteed, by definition, to be nature's opposite. In neither case can we do anything to change this situation."[11] Vogel calls for jettisoning the concept of nature and rewriting environmental theory without it: "[T]he concept of 'nature' might be such an ambiguous and problematic one, so prone to misunderstanding and so riddled with pitfalls, that its usefulness for a coherent environmental philosophy will turn out to be small indeed."[12]

THE NATURE OF CONCEPTS

Vogel accepts this conclusion with no sign of sadness or loss; there is still much to accomplish in environmental theory, he writes, even if logic shows that we must turn our attention from the "natural" world to the world as human habitat. Some other environmentalists agree that nature may be coming to an end but mourn its passing. For them, the problem is not that "nature" is inherently conceptually incoherent but that it is becoming a null set because nature is being humanized in actual fact. Thus, the science journalist Bill McKibben argues that "nature" has been *drained* of its meaning: "We have changed the atmosphere and so we are changing the weather. By changing the weather, we make every spot on earth man-made and artificial. We have deprived nature of its independence, and that is fatal to its meaning. Nature's independence *is* its meaning; without it there is nothing but us."[13] Yet other environmentalists gamely persist in trying to preserve nature. The Sierra Club is still trying to "explore, enjoy, and protect the wild places of the earth"; the Wildlife Conservation Society says it has "the clear mission to save wildlife and wild places across the globe"; and The Nature Conservancy posts under its name the slogan, "Protecting nature. Preserving life."[14] Mill's intractable dilemma is easily stated and attracts scholarly attention; science writers recognize that, as a practical matter, nature is dwindling; and activists may sometimes conclude that their agenda is better fostered by talking about anthropocentric concepts such as public health or outdoor recreation or the benefit of future generations, but many people still want to protect nature. They want to protect the natural world from ever-growing human activity. The question must arise, then, whether the dilemma must be understood quite as starkly as Mill argues: as questions about cows and corn make plain, there is certainly great difficulty in saying exactly what "nature" refers to, but is the bind such that the very idea of nature turns out to be a mirage?

"Nature" in environmentalism must have *something like* the second of Mill's definitions; it has something to do with independence from human doings. But is the independence absolute and rigid? Some see it that way—Vogel and McKibben draw the line very tightly, for instance. Yet McKibben does not draw the line exactly where Vogel (following Mill) does: he does not suppose that the mere presence of any human agency makes a state of affairs no longer natural. He assumes, rather, that the loss of nature results from measurable physical changes to nature and then sets the bar very, very low for deciding what measurable changes transform a "natural" state to an "artifactual" one. And others draw the line higher. John Passmore characterizes the preservationist impulse this way: "By 'preservation' I mean the attempt to maintain in their present condition such areas of the earth's surface as do not yet bear the *obvious* marks of man's handiwork and to protect from the risk of extinction those species of living beings which man has not yet destroyed."[15]

Yet another approach is that taken by Eric Katz, who starts off in Millian fashion by accepting that human agency is always at odds with naturalness. "Once we inject our intentional designs into a natural system, we no longer have a natural system," writes Katz, "we have a garden, a forest plantation, or a farm."[16] Nonetheless, Katz also maintains that a thing can be natural or artifactual to different degrees:

> Naturalness and artifactuality exist along a spectrum of various kinds of entities. Things can be more or less natural, more or less artifactual. A wooden chair is more natural than a plastic chair because it is more closely related to the naturally produced material that forms its basic structure. The plastic chair is farther from its original material or source. But both chairs are definitely artifacts, essentially different from naturally occurring entities, a fallen tree that I sit on while walking through the forest, for example.[17]

The picture Katz gives us seems to be of two properties vying for possession of a thing. The properties themselves are defined purely, but their admixture in actual things can make for more complicated assessments. If the presence of artifactuality is sufficiently great, then the thing overall counts as an artifact; but if only a little artifactuality is present, then the thing might be counted as "natural." As a result, even if the bar for artifactuality is set rather low, the use of the term "natural" need not suppose the complete independence from human agency that Mill's second definition supposes.

The dispute here is not so much about how to define "nature" as about how to use the definition—or what it means to "define" a term, we might say. Mill proposes two definitions of the term "nature" that will tell us precisely what the extension of the concept is, and then he shows that neither definition can be of any use. As actually used, the term does not conform *exactly* to either definition; it is only *close* to one of them. The underlying question is about how concepts like "nature" function. Mill makes a standard philosophical assumption about concepts—namely, that they must have definitions that will clearly adjudicate what it is in the extension of the concept. The actual use of "nature," however, appears to conform better to the account of concepts usually associated with Ludwig Wittgenstein, who held that concepts are understood, not by learning rules for what belongs to the extension of the concept, but by becoming familiar with the extension itself—by learning examples of the concept—and then, secondarily, on the basis of one's knowledge of the examples, gaining insight into the commonalities that knit the concept together. Moreover, the commonalities need not span the entire extension; there might instead be an assortment of characteristics that unite overlapping subsets of the extension. Some members of the extension might lack some traits. And some characteristics might be particularly significant, others less, some important only in combinations. Wittgenstein gave the example of the term "game," which spans a range of uses that have no one thing in common but instead encompass an assortment of similarities and relationships (providing entertainment for participants, providing entertainment for spectators, involving winning and losing, having a definite end, having clearly formulated rules), each of which is characteristic of many, but not all, games. There is, as Wittgenstein said, a family resemblance among the uses; they share similarities and relationships in somewhat the way that related people share traits.[18]

If "nature" works along these lines, then it can refer to a *degree* of independence from human intervention. "Independence," in other words, also need not be defined as absolute freedom from influence and need not provide a bright line with which to sort out "natural" from "artifactual." (And, in fact, that would be a bizarre and impossible understanding of "independence." Who among us is independent in that way? And yet we persist in talking about some people as "independent.") In short, it can sometimes be an open question whether something is natural, not just because we may not be sure about the facts, but because we may not be sure about the word "natural."

A thumbnail account John Passmore gives of how he uses the term provides a quick way into this double-barreled confusion. Passmore explains that he will use the term "so as to include only that which, setting aside the supernatural, is human neither in itself nor in its origins. This is the sense in which neither Sir Christopher Wren nor St Paul's Cathedral forms part of 'nature' and it may be hard to decide whether an oddly shaped flint or a landscape where the trees are evenly spaced is or is not 'natural.'"[19] It can be hard to decide about the stone and the landscape partly for factual reasons, of course: a stone that has been quickly shaped for use as a tool (and then, perhaps, dropped and left alone for some centuries) may look very much like one that has never been touched by a human, and we may simply not know enough about it to decide which it is. But another reason that the decision can be hard is that we may debate the rules of application for the concept. What does it *mean* for something to be human in its "origins"?

McKibben laments that we have changed the atmosphere and made it nonnatural, but surely the atmosphere is not human in its *origins*. Or, suppose we know that a certain stone was used as a tool: we saw someone lift it from the soil, clean it, knock off a projection to create a flat surface on one side, and use it to pound a stake into the ground. Is the stone now an artifact? Surely, the stone is not human in its origins. And is everything that is human in its origins nonnatural? Human feces could reasonably be counted as natural—at least in certain contexts: found in a diaper, they seem natural, but found along a trail while hiking, they may be counted as an intrusion into nature. And, finally, why is it that something "human in itself" is not natural by definition? Maybe humans, like their feces, are nonnatural in some contexts, such as the environmental context that Passmore attends to. But if we are considering what is human in itself *in its own context*—if we are talking about human nature—then we might use "natural" to make distinctions about different ways of treating human nature. We could say that certain things Sir Christopher Wren might have done to himself would not be natural and avoid writing off the person himself as nonnatural.

In short, an adequate explication of "nature" is more likely to involve a long-winded argument than a pat application of any one definition. The further terms with which it is explained—such as "independence" and "origin"—will themselves require interpretation. If it is understood in the open-textured way outlined here, then the way to examine the concept is not to search for some perfectly clear and rigid definition, but to explore the cases. Furthermore, we may discover that "nature" means somewhat different things in different contexts—in environmentalism and in debates about human behavior, for example. It will therefore be necessary to explore it within those contexts. In this chapter, the exploration of nature is only just begun; the basic framework for the exploration is laid down, and the work will have to be carried forward when we turn, later in the book, to some of the debates that involve appeals to nature.

In fact, the argument is more likely to be interminable than merely long-winded. If the term is open-textured and always open to debate, an account of "nature" will, in some sense, never be *completed* once and for all. "Nature" has the characteristics of what W. B. Gallie called *essentially contested* concepts: its rules of application can be variously specified, and no one way of applying it can be proven to be the right way. This prospect, which some will find defeatist, will bring us back to Vogel's suggestion that perhaps we should go forward without "nature," on the grounds that the concept is just too ambiguous and problematic to be useful. But there is no reason to see the essential contestability of "nature" as amounting to a long and inevitable defeat. Many concepts, and perhaps in particular many of the concepts that are important in reaching moral judgments, are understood less than rigidly. For example, there are a handful of terms that are crucial for good moral deliberation but that have so far eluded any widely accepted definition: "person," "adult," "rational," "voluntary," "decisionally incapacitated," "informed consent," "harm," and "benefit." One of the surprises of the history of bioethics has been the difficulty of deciding what "dead" means. In the early 1970s, when the field was just emerging and wading into the clinical encounters between doctors and patients—laying bare and trying to rethink an assortment of seemingly unexamined and unacceptable assumptions and practices among medical professionals—The Hastings Center (where I work, many years later) formed a special task force to address two issues related to death and dying: the definition of death and the decision to forego life support. The assumption was that the definition of death should be sorted out first, making room for the much more difficult problem of deciding when to forego life support. But, almost four decades later, what constitutes death is further from resolution than ever—indeed, there are even more possible answers on the table now than at the start of the debate.[20]

The good news, however, is that the practical questions do not always depend on the definitional questions. Sometimes, undoubtedly, they do: the question about the definition of death raises a problem for some cases of organ transplantation. (Death is sometimes declared on the basis of loss of heart function in order to facilitate organ transplantation; but if death is defined as "irreversible" loss of heart function, and then the stopped heart is extracted and *restarted* in another body, then the condition of "irreversibility" has arguably not been met.) Often, however, the practical questions can be addressed even while definitional uncertainty remains. Harvesting organs can be deemed acceptable even though we are, collectively at least, not quite sure exactly when the person has died. There is also considerable consensus on the practical question of when to stop medical treatment and accept death (whatever exactly it is and whenever exactly it occurs); the persistent uncertainty about whether people are *dead* if they are "brain dead" but on "life support" has complicated but not confounded this debate. Some of the questions about values that bear on decision making at the end of life could be taken up independently. As a series of landmark cases helped establish, a rational adult—or a family member or other person who is close to that person or has been formally designated as a surrogate decision maker—may decide to stop medical treatment even if death has not occurred or is not imminent. Nor do definitional problems with some of these other significant terms—"rational," "adult," or "medical treatment"—completely disable that general principle.

All these terms are contestable yet still serviceable. All admit hard cases, yet we nonetheless communicate with each other adequately well. We carry on. In fact, terms that refer to moral values themselves—"kindness," "cruelty," "generosity," "integrity"—take the definitional fuzziness to still another level, yet we carry on with them, too. In deciding whether the concept of nature is coherent, then, the question is not whether there is some one clear definition of it that lets us sort out every case, but whether it is *serviceable*, in roughly the way that many other morally significant terms are. How the term is applied to the world must be more than smoke, but need not be black and white.

IS "NATURE" NATURAL?

The second problem is that the idea of nature does not correspond to an actually existing reality. Instead, purportedly, "nature" is a cultural and historical phenomenon, alien to many cultures, not even part of Western culture until fairly recently, and always evolving in keeping with the interests of whoever is in power. In philosophical lingo, realism about the concept of nature must give way to constructivism.

Behind this claim, too, lies a long line of careful scholarship, much of it found in the postmodernist theory associated with Jacques Derridas. As Soper puts it, this line invites us "to view the very idea of nature—the idea of that which has standardly been opposed to culture—as itself a cultural formation."[21] It is associated particularly strongly with the romantic movement and its backlash against the industrialization of the nineteenth century. In the United States, it is connected to the transcendentalist movement and, above all, to Henry David Thoreau, whose line "In wildness is the preservation of the world" may well be the most frequently quoted and best remembered of his many epigrams. The aims of these thinkers were often admirable, but—as the postmodern critique has rightly pointed out—the idea of nature that they helped create has often been part of ideologies intended to strengthen and justify oppression and hatred. Again, Soper:

Romantic conceptions of "nature" as wholesome salvation from cultural decadence and racial degeneration were crucial to the construction of Nazi ideology, and an aesthetic of "nature" as source of purity and authentic self-identification has been a component of all forms of racism, tribalism and nationalism. Equally, of course, the appeal to the health, morality, and immutability of what "nature" proposes has been systematically used to condemn the "deviants" and "perverts" who fail to conform to the sexual or social norms of their culture.[22]

Soper calls on environmentalists, who ordinarily deny that the idea of nature is a cultural construction, to use the concept of nature more carefully, "to pay heed to some of the slidings of the signifier that have been highlighted in postmodernist theory."[23] An unthinking and unqualified celebration of nature "can seem insensitive to the emancipatory concerns motivating its rejection."[24] Soper's resolution of this problem is to recommend an ongoing dialectical approach, tacking back and forth between the nature-skepticism of the postmodernists and the nature-endorsement of the environmentalists, taking the claims of both sides seriously but subjecting both to criticism. She hopes thereby to defend a kind of realism about "nature" while always examining claims about nature to ensure that they do not have unjust implications and are not being put to unjust uses.

THE NATURE OF FACTS

Ultimately, Soper's sympathetic discussion of the constructivist critique of nature points not just to a realism that is careful about the implications of its concepts but to a position that combines realism and constructivism. One could hold that nature is a genuinely existing reality *and* that our ways of articulating and delineating it are a matter of cultural convention.

Soper suggests that environmental thought makes use of three different kinds of concepts of "nature." First, "nature" can be understood as a *metaphysical* concept: nature is "the concept through which humanity thinks its difference and specificity. It is the concept of the non-human."[25] Environmentalists tend to suppose (writes Soper) that the distinction between humans and nature must not depend on dualism, that humans and nature must be considered to belong to fundamentally the same kind of reality—a physical reality—but no matter how it is explained on a metaphysical level, a humans–nature distinction of some sort is crucial. Second is a *realist* concept of nature, which refers to "the structures, processes and causal powers that are constantly operative within the physical world, that provide the objects of study of the natural sciences, and condition the possible forms of human intervention in biology or interaction with the environment."[26] The realist concept is what Mill has in mind when he talks about the "powers" of nature and all that takes place through them, and it includes humans. Third is the "lay" or "surface" concept of nature, referring to "ordinarily observable features of the world: the 'natural' as opposed to the urban or industrial environment ('landscape,' 'wilderness,' 'country-side,' 'rurality'), animals, domestic and wild, the physical body in space and raw materials. This is the nature of immediate experience and aesthetic appreciation; the nature we have destroyed and polluted and are asked to conserve and preserve."[27] It is the lay conception, in Soper's account, that is in play when environmentalists define the natural state of affairs that they believe should be protected.

With the lay conception, the "essential point is that we are talking about nature as appearance, and usually of nature as it appears in everyday experience."[28] Soper spends some time looking for some very general marks of nature. Initially, she suggests that the most fundamental contrast that "nature" highlights is that between city and country, but she quickly notes that this cannot be quite right. "Nature" in the lay understanding can be and often is a product of human civilization—the garden and field can be deemed natural. Perhaps (Soper suggests) whether a place can be called "natural" depends in some way on the use and function to which the place is put; if the place plays a vital role in socioeconomic relations, for example, it might be less likely to count as "natural." Soper quotes the French sociologist Henri Lefebvre on this point: "The more a space partakes of nature, the less it enters into the social relations of production."[29] If we are hiking in a remote forest and come across a human structure, our sense of how much the structure damages the naturalness of the forest will vary according to whether it is a cell phone tower or an outhouse.

The key point for the basic problem of whether a realist or a constructivist account of "nature" is preferable is that a "lay" conception of nature is both. On the one hand, it is about an actually existing world: it picks out "ordinarily observable features of the world." As Soper writes, "it is not language that has a hole in its ozone layer."[30] It could be corrected by making new discoveries about the world. We can envision a meteorological discovery that led us to see the hole in the ozone layer as a naturally occurring phenomenon rather than as a result of human agency. On the other hand, the ways in which these states of affairs are demarcated from human affairs is dependent on convention. Which features are picked out, and how they are brought together under the heading "nature," cannot be explained simply by pointing to the world. Soper writes that the garden and the field can be part of the lay concept of nature, for example, but "garden" and "field" could not be explained without reference to convention. And why "garden" and "field" go under the heading "nature" while "empty land where a now razed factory once stood" does not also would require reference to convention. Perhaps, too (although I am straying from Soper's line of thought at this point), a garden or a field would be natural in certain contexts and not in others—next to one's home, as a way of producing food for the dinner table, it might be considered "natural," but stumbled across while hiking in a "wilderness preserve," it might not. The simple fact that humans are *part* of the causal story that explains how a state of affairs came about need not (contrary to McKibben) mean the state of affairs is no longer natural. We must know something more particular about the human causal contribution—how great the human causal contribution is (for example, whether the state of affairs is human in its "origins," as Passmore puts it) and how the human causal contribution is to be interpreted (whether a pile of feces is in a diaper and understood in the context of human development or is found by the side of a trail and understood in the context of a "wilderness").

Suppose that Soper's account of the lay concept of nature is on the right track. Would the convention-dependence of "nature" give reason to dismiss it? It's not clear why that would be so. Facts, in general, are articulated and delineated within the framework of a particular set of shared interests. Mary Midgley has pursued this point: "If someone buys stamps, what is going on can be described as 'buying stamps,' or as the pushing of a coin across a board and the receiving of paper in return—or as a set of muscular contractions—or one of stimulus-response reactions—or a social interaction involving role-playing—or a piece of dynamics, the mere movement of physical masses—or an economic exchange—or a piece of prudence, typical of the buyer. None of these is *the* description."[31] All of these descriptions refer to frameworks of human interests; they are all partly a matter of convention. Facts are "never logically separated from some kind of evaluating,"[32] yet, insofar as they depend on evaluation, they are never merely about the world "out there," independent of human convention.

There are, moreover, other morally significant concepts that refer to the world as it really is yet are framed by social convention. An act is "voluntary," for example, when it is freely chosen. A purist understanding of what it means to choose freely holds that an agent's choice is not determined by external forces; rather, the agent moves himself. This understanding is hard to make sense of, just as a purist understanding of "nature" is. Alternatively, one may hold that all human actions are determined by other forces and that an act counts as "voluntary" when those forces do not amount to social coercion. But, of course, social coercion comes in many flavors. What counts as "social coercion" serious enough to say that a person enduring it is not choosing freely is plainly going to be both subject to empirical arguments and, in part, a matter of convention.

Or consider the related complex term "informed consent" in medical ethics. A patient gives informed consent to a medical intervention when the patient has received adequate information about it, has understood the information, and freely agrees to undergo it. According to the dominant understanding, how much information must be provided, how well it must be understood, and how much confidence there must be to declare that the decision to undergo the intervention is not coerced varies according to the seriousness of the patient's medical situation and the riskiness of the intervention. Again, plainly, much evidenced argument is possible about whether informed consent has been given, *and* these criteria will also be fundamentally a matter of convention.

Finally, consider the virtue of honesty. As with the term "natural," assessing "honesty" requires knowing something about genuine states of affairs in the world. To be honest is, in part, to describe states of affairs *as* they are—not to lie about them. But there is quite a bit more to say about honesty as well. Here's Regina Hursthouse's introductory overview of the virtue in the *Stanford Encyclopedia of Philosophy*:

> An honest person cannot be identified simply as one who…practices honest dealing, and does not cheat. If such actions are done merely because the agent thinks that honesty is the best policy, or because they fear being caught out, rather than through recognising "To do otherwise would be dishonest" as the relevant reason, they are not the actions of an honest person. An honest person cannot be identified simply as one who, for example, always tells the truth, nor even as one who always tells the truth because it *is* the truth, for one can have the virtue of honesty without being tactless or indiscreet. The honest person recognises "That would be a lie" as a strong (though perhaps not overriding) reason for not making certain statements in certain circumstances, and gives due, but not overriding, weight to "That would be the truth" as a reason for making them.[33]

To be honest is not just to describe states of affairs as they are, then, but to do so for the right reasons, at the right times, and in the right way. Nor need a person *always* tell the truth in order to be considered honest. An "honest" person can recognize that other moral considerations sometimes override truth-telling. In addition, most people would probably allow that a basically "honest" person might sometimes have some slips—prevarication, deliberate ambiguity, even occasional outright lies for no particularly good moral reason. In various ways, then, "honesty" is about the world, yet its proper use is also set by convention.

Of course, these various terms are not entirely on all fours with each other, and a thorough analysis might show that they depend on convention in different ways or to different degrees. But this comparison is enough to suggest that we cannot immediately dismiss the concept of nature on grounds that it is a matter of convention. There are other morally significant concepts that refer to the world as it is and whose use is guided by convention.

One significant way that "nature" differs from these terms is that it is not just about the world, but about things in the world that are "independent" of human affairs, and perhaps this makes it seem that the way the *concept itself* works must be independent of human affairs. Rather than just being a human tool developed to understand the world, the rules of application must be handed down from nature, as it were. But this would be a mistake. "Nature" is part of human conceptual schemes just as much as any other concept is.

Another, related difference is that "nature" is sometimes allied to a *metaphysical* distinction between humans and nature and this, too, might give reason to think that the concept cannot be convention dependent. A metaphysical distinction should track categories of being, not matters of human convention. Also, seeing "nature" as allied to a metaphysical distinction would give reason to see it as tracking a sharp, clear line, as Mill supposes it must. A distinction that tracks categories of being would not be bound by the rough and wavering edges of Soper's lay concept of nature.

There is a second aspect to the dismissal of "nature" on grounds that the term is a matter of convention, though, which is that it happened relatively recently. Honesty, by contrast, seems a stable feature of human conceptual schemes and so may be more legitimate. But what should we make of the recency of "nature"? First, we might point out, speaking of nature at all is a feature of our moral attitudes, and it seems unobjectionable that our moral attitudes evolve. Otherwise, we would still endorse slavery and deny female suffrage. Peter Singer has argued that animals have been brought within the "expanding circle" of moral considerability comparatively recently, yet the recency of this change is not thought to pose a special conceptual problem. Perhaps the concern about "nature" is that the very *object* of moral interest has been recently invented—that there was no such *thing* as "nature" before the nineteenth century—but in the account of facts just developed, it is not clear why a changing understanding of what nature is would give a reason to dismiss the concept.

Second, though, there is an important distinction to bear in mind between Soper's "lay conception of nature"—an account that searches for a demarcation of that which is dependent on humanity and that which is reasonably independent of humanity—and an account of nature like that found in romanticism, which attributes special psychological, spiritual, metaphysical, or moral properties to nature. The former makes room for the possibility that there is value in certain ways of treating nature, since only if we can talk about things in the world that are reasonably independent of humanity can it even be possible to say that not everything should be human artifact, that some things should be protected from human interference. The latter relies on special claims about what nature is to establish the importance of having a special relationship to nature. "The stars awaken a certain reverence, because though always present, they are inaccessible; but all natural objects make a kindred impression, when the mind is open to their influence," wrote Emerson.[34] Such thoughts provide an argument for preservationism—and did, when John Muir got hold of them—but it is a very special sort of argument.

The romantic conception of nature is not just a lay conception of nature but also, and maybe more significantly, a metaphysical conception of nature, developed in part to provide a reason for caring morally about the lay conception. It therefore stands or falls independently of the idea that nature can be articulated and delineated in a way that makes it a *possible* object of moral concern. Nor is that idea a new addition to human conceptual schemes. What may be new is the thought that we might want to pay moral attention to it. But this is a change in values, not a creation of a new thing, and changes in values are to be expected.

THE REALMS OF "NATURE"

We need not get rid of any of the general ways in which the term "nature" is used. It has all the various meanings touched on at the start of the chapter. It has Mill's two senses—roughly, "what conforms to the laws of physics" (the meaning intended when the scientific journal *Nature* uses the word as its name) and "what doesn't reflect human agency" (as when scientists try to learn about the behavior of a pride of lions). Also, in addition to the uses in which human behavior is either all in or all out, "nature" is used in middling ways. At one end of a continuum lies what is entirely free of human involvement—most of the universe beyond earth, and the earth as it has been up until 100,000 years or so ago. At the other end lie things whose "origins" seem uncontroversially to be in human invention—big box stores, lunar probes, and the like. Somewhat nearer to the middle, on both sides, lie various other things that most people would readily categorize as either "natural" or "artificial": a stretch of tallgrass prairie maintained with periodic controlled burns and a weedy abandoned lot where a building was recently knocked down.

In these middling uses, usage of the word is guided not by simply looking to see whether a given state of affairs meets the conditions stipulated in a single, clear definition of nature but by applying a rougher understanding of "nature" to a given problem with a given set of interests in mind. It would be too simplistic to assert that the tallgrass prairie is *flatly* natural or nonnatural. Natural with respect to what or in comparison to what? What we should want to say, rather, is that, in the context of a particular point, a strong case could be made that it is natural. As an alternative to a vast manicured lawn or as a way of growing grains (a kind of agriculture), a good case could be made that a tallgrass prairie is appropriately called "natural." A neatly planted straight row of eucalyptus trees provides a more "natural" window view than a high rise, but would be an unnatural intrusion in a "wilderness" park. Chopping down trees also looks to be at odds with the goals of a wilderness park, but it might be quite compatible with organic agriculture. In short, in the middling uses, the term has to be examined in more particular contexts—in the context of environmental preservation, in the context of agriculture, in sports, in human reproduction, in end-of-life medical care, and so on. Usage of the term might vary somewhat across these contexts, and, in some of these contexts, in principle, the term might be less useful than in others.

Consider wind turbines.[35] If we are looking for a simple definition of "natural," wind turbines will be perplexing. A modern wind turbine is an ingenious device; considered strictly in terms of the human ingenuity and effort invested in it, it must be considered well removed from the natural. In some contexts, this will be exactly how we should think of it. My hometown features a museum of science and energy; I can well imagine an exhibit of different strategies humans have developed for powering machines. Somewhere near the beginning of the exhibit would be foot pedals. Modern wind turbines—with a discussion of computer-controlled motors, blade tip speeds, efficiency of electrical generation—would be near the exit. But another way to gauge their "naturalness" is in terms of their effect on the environment. Understood in this context, as an environmental intervention that lessens the human impact on the world, a case could be made for considering them a comparatively "natural" form of energy. Both of these uses of the word rely on empirical facts, but which facts are relevant and how we correlate the use of the word "natural" with those facts are both matters of convention.

Appeals to "nature" are sometimes criticized as misbegotten attempts to recover the "purity" of some imaginary golden age—free of the taint of humanity or of the violations of norms thought to be appropriate to some (possibly imaginary) biological category. (The latter include the sorts of arguments about which Soper cautions us—arguments against homosexuality, against racial marriages, or for the subjugation of one race to another or of women to men, for example.) Sometimes, certainly, nature is invoked for such ends, and we must be on guard against such uses, as Soper advocates. But the account given here of "nature" tends to discourage any idea of purity. Nature need not be entirely distinct from that which is caused by humans, and, although how much or what degree of human agency is compatible with nature is constrained, how the two may be blended is a matter partly of human convention; both of these considerations should discourage us from thinking of nature as pure. The idea that nature means purity stems at least partly from the critics' assumptions about what a definition of "nature" should accomplish. (And although the critics belong to different camps, including postmodernists as well as Mill and his followers, the idea that a definition of "nature" should be pure arguably reflects a scientific perspective. When doing science, nature probably should be defined in an all-or-nothing fashion. And it is interesting to speculate that the view of moral concepts as clearly definable also reflects a broader, scientific way of thinking about morality. We should certainly be scientific about morality in the sense that we should try to understand it accurately, but we should avoid supposing that scientific knowledge provides a model for morality—that terms will be as cleanly defined as they are in science and that judgments will be appraised in the same way as conclusions in science.)

If all this is right, then we must consider in some depth how the term is used in various specific debates about human alteration of nature. Chapter 5 starts in on that, and each of the following chapters will consider the use of "nature" in new contexts and develop new wrinkles in the account of how "nature" may be deployed. The positions developed in chapters five through eight reflect an underlying theoretical commonality—an acceptance of fuzziness and convention-dependence—but they end up reaching somewhat different conclusions about the moral force of concerns about nature and the legitimacy of public policy that takes them up in each context. To get to those conclusions, though, it is necessary first to do some brush-clearing on the other philosophical problems that concerns about nature put on the table.

NOTES

1. Kate Soper, *What Is Nature? Culture, Politics, and the Non-Human* (Oxford, U.K.: Blackwell, 1995), 1.
2. Mark Sagoff, "Genetic Engineering and the Concept of the Natural," in *Genetic Prospects: Essays on Biotechnology, Ethics, and Public Policy*, ed. V. V. Gearing (Oxford, U.K.: Rowman & Littlefield, 2003), 27–35, at 28.

3. J. S. Mill, "Nature," in *Essential Works of John Stuart Mill* (New York: Bantam Books, 1961), 370.
4. Ibid., 374.
5. Ibid.
6. Ibid., 381.
7. Bonnie Steinbock, "The Appeal to Nature," in *The Ideal of Nature: Debates about Biotechnology and the Environment* (Baltimore, Md.: Johns Hopkins University Press, 2011), 98–113, at 98.
8. J. S. Mill, *Principles of Political Economy*, vol. 2 (London: John Parke, 1848), p. 311; quoted in David Wiggins, "Nature, Respect for Nature, and the Human Scale of Values," *Proceedings of the Aristotelian Society* 100 (2000), 1–32. The passage is also discussed by Bonnie Steinbock, to whom I am indebted for locating it; "The Appeal to Nature," 110.
9. President's Commission for the Study of Ethical Problems in Medicine and Biomedical and Behavioral Research, *Splicing Life: A Report on the Social and Ethical Issues of Genetic Engineering with Human Beings* (Washington, D.C.: President's Commission for the Study of Ethical Problems in Medicine and Biomedical and Behavioral Research, 1982), 55.
10. Ibid., 56–57.
11. Steven Vogel, "Why 'Nature' Has No Place in Environmental Philosophy," in *The Ideal of Nature: Debates about Biotechnology and the Environment* (Baltimore, Md.: Johns Hopkins University Press, 2011), 84–97, at 87.
12. Ibid., 96.
13. Bill McKibben, *The End of Nature* (New York: Random House, 1989), 58.
14. The Sierra Club, "Sierra Club Policies," http://www.sierraclub.org/policy/; Wildlife Conservation Society, "About Us," http://www.wcs.org/about-us.aspx; The Nature Conservancy, http://www.nature.org/.
15. John Passmore, *Man's Responsibility for Nature: Ecological Problems and Western Traditions*, 1st ed. (New York: Charles Scriber's Sons, 1974), 101, italics added.
16. Eric Katz, "Preserving the Distinction between Nature and Artifact," in *The Ideal of Nature: Debates about Biotechnology and the Environment* (Baltimore, Md.: Johns Hopkins University Press, 2011), 71–83, at 73.
17. Ibid., 75.
18. Ludwig Wittgenstein, *Philosophical Investigations*, 3rd ed., tr. G. E. M. Anscombe (Englewood Cliffs, N.J.: Prentice Hall, 1958), sections 66, 67.
19. Passmore, *Man's Responsibility for Nature*, 207. Quoted in Soper, *What Is Nature?*, 16.
20. Robert M. Veatch, "The Evolution of Death and Dying Controversies," *Hastings Center Report* 39, no. 3 (2009): 16–19.
21. Soper, *What Is Nature?*, 7.
22. Ibid., 32.
23. Ibid., 9.
24. Ibid., 8.
25. Ibid., 155.
26. Ibid., 155–56.
27. Ibid., 156.
28. Ibid., 181.
29. Ibid., 185.
30. Ibid., 151.

31. Mary Midgley, *Beast and Man: The Roots of Human Nature* (London, U.K.: Routledge Classics, 2002), 5–6, italics mine.
32. Ibid., 180.
33. Regina Hursthouse, "Virtue Ethics," *Stanford Encyclopedia of Philosophy*, first published July 18, 2003; revised July 18, 2007; http://plato.stanford.edu/entries/ethics-virtue/.
34. Ralph Waldo Emerson, "Nature," in *Essays and Poems by Ralph Waldo Emerson* (New York: Barnes and Noble Classics, 2004), 11.
35. The example is drawn from Christopher Preston, "Synthetic Biology: Drawing a Line in Darwin's Sand," *Environmental Values* 17 (2008): 23–39, at 26.

CHAPTER 2

Perceptions of the Soul

The Nature of Morality

If we can get a serviceable understanding of what, in a given context, a "natural" state of affairs would be, then a second perplexing question arises: why should we value nature? One answer to this question will be uncontested: nature will sometimes be valuable because it helps us obtain something else that is valuable. But this answer will not always get us as far as we might want, since there are some things in nature that people value but that are very unlikely ever to be useful, and the fact that they are *useful* feels beside the point. The problem is answering the question: why should we ever value nature in and of itself—why should nature ever be considered intrinsically valuable?

The microbiologist Lee Silver formulates a version of this question in his book *Challenging Nature*, following a description of a trip to Peru to catch a glimpse of some of the last remaining giant otter:

> I decided to challenge the group with an impertinent question: "Why should we care if the giant otter species goes extinct?" I saw a silent look of horror on everyone's face. How could I pose such a question, they wondered, to this group of people in this place? Attempts were made at providing rational explanations, but none were truly compelling. Like many other widely shared attitudes toward Mother Nature, the idea that we should care just feels right, although people don't quite know why.[1]

Is the human extirpation of animal and plant species, or even the destruction of entire ecosystems, worth caring about morally, in and of itself?

Similarly, why should anybody care whether food is "natural" or not (as long as it is nutritious and its production is economically beneficial), and why should anybody care whether human nature is substantially changed by emerging biotechnologies?

Silver believes that the valuation of nature amounts to a kind of superstitious voodoo. Other critics, usually not quite as harsh, still find in it something irrational and emotional. I will argue in this chapter that the criticism is not entirely off the mark: the best way of explaining why anybody should care about nature probably starts by saying that moral concern about nature is a partly emotional phenomenon. But the criticism does not call attention to a special problem with moral concern with nature. I shall suggest, in fact, that all moral stances are emotional phenomena in the same way and that, even if we understand moral stances as emotional phenomena, we need not regard them as irrational. To nail down this last claim, however, I shall have to allow that there are different ways in which emotions can influence reasoning. A purely emotional approach to morality would also be a contradiction in terms; to engage in moral deliberation is to step back from one's immediate reaction and think critically about it. If we relied unquestioningly on our initial feelings about a moral problem, much that we count as moral progress would not have occurred. Scrutiny must be possible.

WHAT MATTERS

The problem facing those who care about nature is that the going theories of morality in the Western philosophical tradition tend to locate moral value only in aspects of consciousness. Theorists in the Aristotelian tradition tend to hold that moral value consists in the attainment of human well-being, understood to consist in exercise of the virtues combined with such goods as pleasure, intellectual understanding, friendship, and honor. Those in the utilitarian tradition hold that happiness, understood as a state that requires some degree of cognitive activity, is the moral lodestone: what contributes to happiness is good. Kantians hold that moral value consists in the ability to conform to the moral law, understood itself to be a product of reason. How, then, can we explain why mere *nature* can have intrinsic value? It seems to be morally neutral.

One answer sometimes given to this problem in bioethics draws on the natural law tradition and holds that nature is an ultimate *source* of moral guidance. How we ought to treat human beings, that is, can be determined by actually looking to how human beings naturally *are*. Leon Kass is often thought to hold this view, and many proponents of technologies to enhance human beings consider Kass their primary opposition (although how best to interpret Kass and what specifically must be said about human nature in order to have intrinsic misgivings about human enhancement are questions I shall pick up again in Chapter 8). This kind of view would require a robust philosophical defense, as it makes a strong and, on its face, not intuitively plausible claim about the importance of nature; it was this kind of view that Mill had in his sights in his broadside "On Nature."

So the trick is to figure out how to avoid the problem Mill attacks while endorsing Mill's dismay in contemplating a world in which "the spontaneous activity of Nature" is dramatically rolled back by human improvement of it—with "scarcely a place left where a wild shrub or flower could grow without being eradicated in the name of improved agriculture."[2] The problem of nature's intrinsic value has accrued a long commentary in environmental philosophy. Partly, maybe, this is because the philosophical problem looks particularly severe there, since the environment can be assimilated to the usual explanations of moral value less easily than human or animal nature. Partly, maybe, it is because the *practical* problem looks particularly severe: we have had a hundred-plus years now to think about the human ability to make rapid, dramatic, and more or less permanent changes to the environment. Human nature and animal nature are also undoubtedly changed by human behavior, but some of these effects have been with us so long that they look like familiar phenomena. Partly, undoubtedly, the attention to this topic in environmental philosophy is due to the fact that moral concern about the environment is widespread; the idea that the environment deserves moral concern has acquired the status of a settled judgment (hence the silent horror when Silver questioned it), and the problem is how to explain it. For all these reasons, attitudes toward the environment provide a kind of base case for thinking about the moral status of human modification of nature.

One strategy for explaining the value of nature has been to work on the links between nature and the things that the Western philosophical canon already accepts as valuable. For example, Bernard Rollin has argued that the value people find in nature is aesthetic, not moral, but that because finding beauty in the world makes people happy, others should treat that reaction with respect and preserve what makes it possible.[3] Thomas Hill has suggested that whereas nature cannot have moral value, an attitude of respect toward nature might be morally important because it is a sign of a good character.[4] Both of these explanations of appeals to nature are indirect: nature does not itself have moral value, but preserving nature may promote other things that do have moral value. For many environmental philosophers, however, the indirect strategy seems to come up shy of the mark. Efforts to protect sea turtles or old growth forests are rooted in a belief that causing the extinction of sea turtles or the elimination of all old growth forests would be a bad thing in itself, not bad only because it would promote some other bad thing.

The other general strategy, then, is to show that nature itself has moral value. Some environmental philosophers have developed a very strong version of this position: they have tried to establish that nature has value even if nobody actually values it. The reason people *can* find value in nature is that the value is literally *there*, waiting to be found.[5] In effect, the moral value of a natural item is just another property that the item possesses, alongside its colors and shapes and so on. A claim like this requires an elaborate metaphysical system, however, to show how value can be "part of the fabric of the universe," as philosophers sometimes say. Arne Naess, for example, proposes that the relations between entities are partly constitutive of the entities themselves, so that even such seemingly subjective properties as that of "being melancholic," although ascertainable only to valuers, can nonetheless be real features of the world.[6]

Mostly, these positions have not won many adherents, though. A more modest strategy, with less metaphysical baggage, is to hold that natural states of affairs have moral value (in the strong sense that they are valued for themselves rather than as a means to some other value), but that their moral value is always imputed to them, never just discovered in them. This strategy has been developed by the environmental philosopher J. Baird Callicott. It would provide no solution if the value of nature was unique in this respect, but Callicott offers the claim within a broader theory of moral value: he holds that nothing has value in any stronger sense; the value things have—whether human happiness or reason—is always only imputed to them.

This is the view associated with the empiricist philosopher David Hume, who held that moral judgments are rooted in the "passions." This was a technical term for Hume, which is important to bear in mind, since to a contemporary reader the term is easily mistaken for something like "feelings of infatuation or excitement." By "passions," Hume meant a "perception of the mind" that arises in the "soul"—that is, deeply and maybe ineradicably within oneself (Hume was skeptical that there was an immortal soul separate from the body). He distinguished passions from the perceptions he called "ideas," which arise from operations of reason alone, and from immediate sense impressions.[7]

Consider willful murder, Hume says: the act itself is simply a series of movements. No empirical investigation will reveal the values at stake in it, and no train of logic will show what the relevant values are. To find the value, we have to look not to the world, but to our attitudes toward the world: "You never can find [the vice], till you turn your reflexion into your own breast, and find a sentiment of disapprobation, which arises in you, towards this action."[8] Similarly, why should we care about happiness, or honesty, or justice? Not, according to the Humean analysis, because we can discern that those values actually reside in states of affairs in the world independent of human apprehension of them—waiting, as it were, to be discovered by someone with the right investigative tools—but rather because they are deeply entrenched in human ways of apprehending and responding to the world. They are deeply important to us.

This problem—the difficulty of showing why a state of affairs should be valued or disvalued simply by investigating the thing itself—is what has come to be known as the "is-ought" problem. No investigation of what the thing *is* will show how we *ought* to respond to it. Within bioethics, the "is-ought" problem is frequently thought to refer to a narrower problem—namely, the difficulty of showing why we should value that which merely happens to be. Thus, the is-ought problem is frequently trotted out precisely to counter the idea that we can legitimately value *natural* states of affairs. But the real target of the is-ought problem is much broader: it shows not only that we cannot prove the value of nature, but that we cannot prove the value of *any* state of affairs, even those that are accepted in the Western canon, because we cannot get behind our values in the necessary way. Why should we value human happiness? Why should we value rationality and the observance of the duties that reason perhaps reveals to us? At the end of the day, not much more can be said than that we just do.

Many people, writes Simon Blackburn, a prominent contemporary philosopher who defends the Humean account of values, feel that the account "smells of sulphur." The account "is thought of as skeptical, or relativistic, or somehow slightly less than fully respectful of the awful majesty of ethical thought."[9] I have shared this reaction myself at times. If the account is carefully developed, however, it can be deeply sensitive to the richness and complexity of moral thinking. But articulating it is a delicate matter. Slightly overemphasizing one or another aspect of it, in a way that makes the whole account seem a little off, is very easy. The word "emotion" is particularly vexing. One must guard against endorsing "emotivism," an early twentieth-century position that draws on Hume's position but that presents moral emotions dismissively, as a more or less formless slop, and implies that moral judgments are of lesser status than empirical or logical statements. In this account, moral judgments are *merely* feelings. To make a moral judgment that one ought not commit murder is only to say, in effect, "Murder: boo!" This is not Hume's position. Hume spent much time describing various kinds of typical moral responses and how they relate to each other, ending up with a kind of taxonomy of the virtues. His goal is not at all to show that moral judgments are second-class citizens among human utterances, and he does not think his account of them should dislodge their hold on us. "Those who have denied the reality of moral distinctions," he notes at the start of the *Enquiry Concerning Human Understanding*, are "disingenuous disputants." No one "could ever seriously believe, that all characters and actions are alike entitled to the affection and regard of everyone." The only way of converting such an antagonist is to leave him alone, for "it is probable he will, at last, of himself, from mere weariness, come over to the side of common sense and reason."[10] Hume's point is not that morality is silly or unimportant, but only that logic and empirical investigation alone cannot generate moral judgments. In effect, morality is itself, for Hume, a matter of human nature.

To be sure, Hume tends to describe moral disagreements as coming rather quickly to a blunt declaration that what recommends a position is either a "feeling of pleasure or agreeableness" or a contrasting feeling of "disagreeableness." Moral discussions might then seem to reduce quickly to crude battering—one person asserting, "It seems good to me," the other, "Not to me it doesn't." But there could, in fact, be quite a lot to say about a position. A sophisticated modern Humean is likely to speak of something like attitudes, stances, concerns, or stable and considered desires instead of "sentiments" or "passions," to convey that we are dealing not with fleeting whims or raw urges but with a considered and stable aspect of character, and then to observe that attitudinal stances are incorporated in language in so-called "thick" terms such as kindness, generosity, candor, and friendship. "Thick" in this context means that a good explanation of these terms and how they are used requires a lot of concrete description, with examples and qualifications. As the description builds up, and as new terms are described, one would end up working toward a rich anthropological study of the culture in which they are used. When using thick words, then, moral disputants are not forced to talk vaguely about what "feels right" to them; they must go in the exact opposite direction. They must try to articulate those feelings and position them within a cultural framework.[11]

In short, there need be no phenomenological divide between a sophisticated Humean account of moral value and at least one form of moral "realism"—that is, a moral metaethical theory according to which moral judgments can be true or false because they reflect how things actually stand in the world. As John McDowell, David Wiggins, Sabina Lovibond, and some others have argued[12] (drawing on Aristotle, Ludwig Wittgenstein, and Donald Davidson, and—in bioethics—inspiring Hilde Lindemann, James Nelson, and Carl Elliott, among others[13]), evaluative stances can themselves be part of the world if we acknowledge that we cannot separate out reality, thought, and language as if they were separate but parallel systems. We think about reality only by means of language. Since language is fundamentally evaluative, however, nothing bars us from affirming that evaluative stances are *real*, as long as there is sufficient agreement on the correct use of the term. This condition does not hold for "thin" moral terms such as "good" or "right," since there is little agreement on correct application of those terms, but it plausibly can hold for rich or "thick" moral terms such as "honest," "kind," "conscientious," or "discreet"—terms that have an ineliminable evaluative component but have complex yet recognizable patterns of correct use.

Thus, this realist account looks very much like a sophisticated, Blackburn-style Humean account—an account that Blackburn calls "quasi-realist." For starters, both tend to emphasize that moral deliberation is best anchored in thick moral language rather than in thin terms like "good" or "right," both encourage one to suppose that moral thinking and moral discussion will be a complex social phenomenon rather than primarily a rational application of moral principles (since those principles are about what is good or right), and both allow that reality includes evaluative stances. Where they differ is chiefly in how they understand evaluative stances to be part of reality. The realist supposes that it is impossible to get behind the evaluative component of our concepts and talk about reality as being free of values. The quasi-realist says that we can talk about the world prior to or independent of our projection onto it of values, so that we might as well say we live in a value-free world, but that *valuing things* is very much part of reality—a part of human nature that we cannot deny and need not be embarrassed about.

Going forward, it is worth bearing in mind that the realist position remains available, but I shall be satisfied with the quasi-realist position—the sophisticated Humean account. As I shall argue in the remainder of this chapter, it is elegant, it fits with other positions we are likely to want to endorse, and it squares nicely with the lived experience of morality—but for those who feel that it does not do justice to the majesty of ethical thought, that moral judgments simply must be grounded on more than human desire, I think the realist position will capture much of what I present in following chapters. Both positions also allow that the range of things that can be valued is broader than just happiness or obedience to moral duties as revealed by reason: both present moral judgments as a matter of human response to states of affairs in the world (in the realist case, a response that is tantamount to mastery of relevant moral concepts and, in the Humean case, a response that reflects mastery of the relevant concepts).

Thus, as Callicott argues, we may have moral responses to natural states of affairs, just as we can to human states of affairs.[14] Value can be imputed to other species, to ecosystems. Blackburn makes the point, too:

> Consider as well such problems as expressing genuine respect for the wilder-nesses of the world, or for the diversity of living species, except in unconvincing terms about how useful they are, for example as sources of medicine. Here we need to find a moral force behind respect for the independence, or grandeur, or sublime nature of the wilderness, although we find it difficult to do so without sounding sentimental or romantic. But take the actual case in which an adver-tising concern hatched the plan of putting a disk into space, about the apparent size of the moon, on which advertising slogans and images would be generated, thereby becoming compulsory and permanent sights in the night sky. It is hard in conventional terms to show that anyone is "harmed" by such a project.... And doubtless some people would *like* it. Yet it is not over-delicate to see the proposal as disgusting, a violation, a symptom of a break in the tie between humanity and the cosmos, an outrage against the dignity of the natural order of things.[15]

Similarly, value could be found in aspects of human lives that are not sim-ply aspects of human consciousness: perhaps to the fact that humans are sexual creatures, to the chance recombinations of genes by which people come into being, or to the diversity of bodies in which we have our being, even to human finitude. In discussing cloning, for example, Kass expounds evocatively on sexual reproduction's commingling of the parents' genetic lines, its connection to sexuality and marriage, its chanciness and lack of full parental control. "In natural procreation," wrote President George W. Bush's President's Council on Bioethics (in language that presumably owes more than a little to Kass), "two individuals give life to a new human being whose endowments are not shaped deliberately by human will, whose being remains mysterious, and the open-endedness of whose future is rati-fied and embraced."[16] In none of this is there a logically compelling account of why we *must* value sexuality. But, for some people, it will be enough to establish that we *do*—or at least, that they do. By reminding us of the many surprises of having children and the mysteries and thrills of watching them develop, coaxing them along, and inevitably letting go of them, the Council hopes to elicit from us a sense of something so special and wonderful about natural human procreation that losing it is a moral loss.

In a widely ridiculed article in *The New Republic*, Kass asserted that a visceral emotional reaction may sometimes provide moral guidance. "In crucial cases," wrote Kass, "...repugnance is the emotional expression of deep wisdom, beyond reason's power fully to articulate it."[17] We may be repelled by the use of cloning to produce children, for example, "because we intuit and feel, immediately and without argument, the violation of things we rightfully hold dear." Such language led to a derisive profile of Kass in *The American Prospect*, titled "Irrationalist in Chief," which slammed the "Wisdom of Repugnance" as "a grand piece of anti-intellectualism" and a "pseudo-intellectual defense of 'yuck' reactions."[18] The Humean account of how we find value in human nature would be one way of understanding Kass's line that "we intuit and feel" the violation of things we hold dear. (It is not the only way of understanding Kass's position, however, and it might not be an approach that Kass himself would endorse.) More must be said about the idea that we feel a violation of our values "immediately and without argument," of course. In the Humean account, a moral judgment is immediate in that it is a response directly to states of affairs in the world, and it is "without argument," in that it cannot be justified by some further consideration. Moral judgments are neither immediate nor without argument in another sense. I shall delve further into this point later. First, however, I want to offer some additional observations about what makes the Humean account philosophically attractive.

PHILOSOPHICAL MODESTY
AND THEORETICAL SKEPTICISM

Ascribing value to states of nature is often thought to require wooly philosophical reasoning that either makes great, unjustified leaps or involves many intricate steps that are eye-glazingly difficult to follow and well outside the central lines of philosophical and scientific thought. Hume's view of morality is not merely not wooly, however, but streamlined, elegant, and compatible with other well-accepted lines of thought. Here are four large advantages it enjoys:

Modesty

First, defending it requires no philosophical extravagances. One need not show how practical reason can loop reflexively back onto itself to generate what Kant called an "end-in-itself"; nor why, if a person values her own happiness, she must also, as a matter of reason, equally value other people's happiness; nor how values can be real features of the world. One need not posit the existence of a natural moral law that inheres in the cosmos and is apprehensible to all rational beings (what Jeremy Bentham called "nonsense on stilts"). Nor need one elaborately circumnavigate the is-ought divide; on the contrary, this position takes that divide as a starting point.

I do not mean to suggest that the Humean account is free of metaphysics and philosophical assumptions while opposing positions are embroiled in them. Every account of moral values must include an account of what moral values *are*—what their standing is, what kind of compulsion they generate, and how they are justified. The Humean metaphysics are just rather elegant and uncomplicated and fit well with much else that is accepted about the world today.

Comprehensiveness and Unity

Second, Hume's account can give us something to say about all aspects of morality and moral reasoning, starting off with the bedrock questions about what moral values and moral judgments are. Much work in bioethics arguably shelves these questions. Indeed, perhaps this has always been part of the appeal of bioethics. Part of what has often seemed helpful about Tom Beauchamp and James Childress's *Principles of Biomedical Ethics* is that it suggests practical bioethics can begin where philosophical speculation about the nature of moral commitments leaves off.[19] Beauchamp and Childress offer principles that may be supported from a variety of different theoretical frameworks. That is all well and good, as long as we really are largely agreed on our normative moral principles. Disagreements about what we do to human nature suggest that we are not.

Hume's account also explains how moral insight leads to action in a comprehensible and straightforward way: if to reach a moral judgment is to react emotionally, then we can say that a person does not genuinely understand what "cruelty" is (for example) unless she has a visceral response when she sees an instance of it: to see cruelty is to experience a turning of the gut, a surge of anger, and to be moved to do something about it. Many have thought that having such reactions is part and parcel of really understanding a moral concept like "cruelty," and Hume's account accommodates this thought very easily. By contrast, if a moral judgment is fundamentally a rational recognition, however, then a little fancy footwork is required to show that the judgment is internally connected to the right emotional responses.

Fit with a Scientific World View

What Callicott seems most to like about Hume's account is how well it fits into a scientific world view. Scientists, Callicott points out, also tend to begin with a sharp distinction between fact and value. "From the scientific point of view, nature throughout, from atoms to galaxies, is an orderly, objective, [value-neutral] domain. Value is, as it were, projected onto natural objects or events by the subjective feelings of observers."[20]

Hume's account is particularly congenial to the world view of biologists, Callicott argues, because it can be connected with evolutionary theory.[21] Darwin thought that a capacity for sympathy would give members of a social species a survival advantage because it makes for better, more committed parenting and more tight-knit and supportive social groups. Some recent theorists have streamlined this view by arguing that selection operates not on organisms but on genes and that genes might be more likely to perpetuate themselves if the organisms carrying them have innate tendencies to support and defend other organisms that carry the same genes. Some will find this reductionist account of morality unsatisfying, but other recent theorists have sought to broaden and complicate it. Paul Ehrlich has argued, for example, that instead of seeing morality as filling specific purposes—promoting cooperation, discouraging infighting—we can see it as part of a broader capacity that humans evolved to create systems of meaning by which they could communicate with each other and organize themselves.[22] Humans evolved to be culture-creating organisms, but cultures take on an evolutionary life of their own, and, although they may sometimes give a species a survival advantage, they may also acquire traits that are disadvantageous. They may even sometimes become dangerous and self-destructive.

The Humean need not choose from among the different versions of the evolutionary account of morality; Hume himself took the existence of moral sentiments simply as a given—a feature of the creatures we happen to be. That these accounts are available, making morality itself a topic of scientific investigation, is an appealing feature of Hume's account, however.

Fit with Everyday Moral Language

A fourth advantage of Hume's account is that it also squares well with our everyday experience of morality. A preliminary point to note here is that the Humean account fits less well than some other theories with the idea that moral judgments can justifiably be called "true" or "false"—and that this is an argument in favor of the theory. Reasonable, thoughtful people are more likely to evince a kind of moral humility, an openness to alternative views, than they are to trumpet a position as "true" or to blow it away as being "false." In everyday conversation, people mostly do not speak of "truth" when it comes to moral judgments. We tend to speak instead of "views" or "positions."

To be sure, Blackburn argues that moral judgments can be reckoned true or false, at least if we invoke only a kind of bare-bones conception of truth: if a statement *p* is true if and only if *p*—for example, if it is true that beating one's children is wrong if and only if beating one's children is wrong—then nothing stands in the way of saying that it is true that beating one's children is wrong.[23] (Blackburn's way of claiming truth susceptibility for moral judgments is not very different from how realists such as McDowell or Wiggins claim truth susceptibility for moral judgments.[24]) Blackburn is perhaps reaching here; the everyday phenomenology seems to lean away from "truth" assignment, and other Humeans shy away from this claim. Bernard Williams, for example, assumes that truth can appropriately be imputed to statements only in fields where there is evidence that, over time, drives people to reject some statements and accept others.[25] In other words, truth is predicable only within fields in which people tend to *converge* on a set of positions and the convergence is *explained* by evidence. Moral judgments are very different in this way from, say, facts about geography. Certainly we endorse, accept, evaluate, waffle over, depart from, and reject moral judgments, but it is hard to show that we make those moves for the same kinds of reasons that we endorse, accept, evaluate, waffle over, depart from, and reject claims about the world. One cannot imagine ever learning that one was wrong about abortion in the same way that one could learn one was wrong about where Tanzania is.[26]

The Humean account also fits well with the kinds of values we are likely to invoke when thinking about a case and the way we are likely to argue about a judgment. I shall say more later about what moral argument looks like in the Humean account. But think for a moment about the kinds of value terms that come into play in actual moral debate. When we think and talk about what we ought to do—when we are in the midst of a problem, that is, not when we are at repose in an armchair—we tend not to start in with theoretic constructs like autonomy or utility. Instead, we bring up the thick terms—everyday moral notions like kindness, honor, integrity, conscientiousness, loyalty, humility, respectfulness, responsibility, and the like. Hume's account can accommodate this fact well.

Stressing this point helps distinguish a sophisticated Humean position from the simplistic emotivism of early twentieth-century moral philosophy.

Emotivism offered an account of the meaning of value words; its characteristic thesis was that to say something is good is simply to endorse it and to say something is bad is simply to indicate disapproval—"Murder: boo!" Emotivism was really an attempt to explain morality away—to leave it out of a scientific world view. But Hume's account does not commit us to this agenda. To the contrary, it can help us take on the ethical life in all its complexity.

A rich, true-to-life moral language appears in some respects less powerful and in other respects more powerful than the substitute theoretical language of moral philosophy. On the one hand, because it roots moral deliberation in a heterogeneous web of commitments and interests, it may seem to lead to less rigorous moral deliberation. On the other hand, it allows us to capture distinctions between different sorts of moral reactions that are lost if they must be cashed out in the common coin of autonomy or utility. One is able to say, for example, that sex with children is repugnant and horrifying (not merely that it is a violation of children's autonomy and might harm them) and that redemptive love is beautiful (not merely that it is especially utility maximizing). Also, of course, one might be able to say such things as that sex with dead bodies or with animals is repugnant or that embryos are not morally equivalent to either skin tissue or full-grown adults—points that are pretty much without footing if one must appeal to moral notions rooted, as autonomy and utility are, in claims about human consciousness.

Thus, the move to a Humean account of moral valuation both introduces and deemphasizes moral theory: it introduces some questions about the nature of value (the topic of metaethics), but sets aside—or at least pushes to the background—efforts to show how moral judgments fall out of first principles about, say, autonomy and utility (which have to do with normative ethics). This is another example of its philosophical modesty. Perhaps we could say that one respect in which it is immodest is with respect to the question of what kinds of values can legitimately come into play in moral thinking: it lets in more of our everyday language. But the burden of proof is on those who think the broad, familiar range of value terms people actually use needs to be replaced by a more rigidly ordered kind of moral deliberation.

SUBJECTIVISM AND RELATIVISM

In a nutshell, part of the argument for the Humean account is the easy explanation it gives us of the ontological standing of moral judgments. Criticism of the Humean account centers on some implications it seems to

have for the *social* standing of moral judgments. It seems—to many people—to imply that moral judgments are not as authoritative as we would
like to say they are. But, I shall argue, there is much to say to allay this
concern. When we are discussing the ontology of values, simplicity is a virtue, but when we turn to the sociology of moral judgments, complexity is
a virtue.

Perhaps the most important concern is that Hume's account appears to
commit one to subjectivism and therefore also to relativism—to holding,
that is, that moral judgments are entirely a person's own views and therefore that they hold only for a given person or perhaps for a given culture, if
the culture is sufficiently homogenous. People have different feelings, after
all; how can any one feeling be "correct"?

Of course, relativism of a sort may well be appropriate: although we
might want to maintain that certain core commitments hold for all people
and cultures, we could still acknowledge relativism about *how* one shows
respect. Depending on the culture, one might need to remove one's hat or
keep it on, or remove one's shoes, or avoid showing the soles of the shoes,
and so on. But the complaint about Hume's account is that it seems to
allow relativism even about commitments that we hold most dear because
other people might hold other commitments dear, and we have no way of
deciding which commitments are ultimately the right ones.

If the complaint is framed just like that—as a complaint that Hume's
account cannot sort out the ultimate moral truth—then it has merit. But
here's what can be said in favor of Hume's account: it does not compel us to
let everyone cling to their own moral judgments no matter how wrong we
believe them to be. Our moral commitments are (only!) about what matters most to us. Because they cannot be derived from or judged by anything
that lies outside morality, we need not suspend moral deliberation to see
whether our commitments are ultimately defensible. Indeed, we are unable
to do that. As Blackburn writes, "it is only by using our sensibilities that we
judge value."[27] If we are committed to our commitments, then we need not
relinquish them just because somebody else disagrees with us.

Furthermore, our sensibilities can allow us to render judgments about
other lives and cultures. This means, argues Bernard Williams, that it is
always either too early or too late for relativism: it is too early when the
members of a culture have never met another culture and thought of "an
alternative to 'us'.... It is too late, when they confront the new situation,
that requires them to see beyond their existing rules and practices."[28]
Perhaps the point could be put most powerfully this way: one's moral views
are so much a part both of one's identity and of one's view of the world
that it is impossible either to suspend them or to delimit their scope, as is

necessary if they are merely relative to a social context. Indeed, as noted in Chapter 1, we cannot even identify "facts" without using our values, as Mary Midgley (although she is not a Humean) reminds us. A given fact can always be described in a variety of different ways, broken down into multiple other "facts" or lumped into other larger ones. In a given interaction between two people, psychologists, sociologists, biologists, physicists, and artists will individuate various sets of facts, and which description we use will depend on what our interests are at the moment. But if facts are "never logically separated from some kind of evaluating,"[29] then it is impossible to see morality as reaching only so far.

Relativism is a challenge, of course, for any account of morality that does not represent morality as fundamentally mistaken and senseless. If we try to derive moral judgments from an account of human flourishing, for example, then we are compelled to argue against relativism by defending our account of human flourishing against rival possibilities. Hume's account sets us in the other direction, by eliminating this search for foundations. If we insist on trying to make sense of "moral truth," then we will do so by saying that a moral judgment is "true" if and only if it is one that really should be endorsed, which is simply to say that it genuinely reflects our moral attitudes. There is no requirement that it square with the world as it can be understood independent of our moral attitudes. Thus, Blackburn holds, "There is no problem of relativism because there is no problem of moral truth. Since moral opinion is not in the business of representing the world, but of assessing choices and actions and attitudes in the world, to wonder which attitude is right is to wonder which attitude to adopt or endorse."[30]

Perhaps these observations will also help head off another, related complaint: we want moral principles to be universal laws. The relativism challenge is aimed ostensibly at the prospect of losing universality, but it may be that losing the feeling of having laws imposed on us is the more alarming prospect. If moral judgments arise out of the emotions, instead of from reason, then they do not seem to be *enforced*; they seem to be optional, contingent. And then maybe the candle is not worth the game; fully accepting the Humean account will undermine the very phenomenon it tries to account for.[31] Or so goes this complaint. But why would one stop caring about what one genuinely cares about? And how would one do it? Only by invoking other things we care about.

Sometimes, of course, reflecting on our moral views may lead us to believe that we have been mistaken, and we may sometimes come to see another viewpoint as valuable. But this is only to recognize that travel broadens the mind, as Blackburn puts it. Relativism is not yet established, only reassessment. And to reassess, we must engage with our moral values—reaffirming them, sometimes modifying them, or perhaps even abandoning some view we have held.

It is such mind-broadening that Erik Parens urges on us about the issue of human enhancement. Parens describes the debate over new enhancement biotechnologies as pitting two "psycho-ethical frameworks" against each other: enthusiasts about enhancement technologies stand for the self-creativity that those technologies help make possible, whereas critics stand for a sense of gratitude for having been created—"for the mysterious whole, which we have not made"—and so worry that enhancement technologies will undermine that gratitude.[32] Parens holds that most thoughtful, honest people will acknowledge, when they consider their intuitions about a range of cases, that both of these frameworks have some hold on them, to one degree or another. Thus, for Parens, questions about what can be done to enhance or "normalize" human bodies and behaviors are caught in some indeterminacy: most people, for at least some cases, simply do not have overwhelmingly strong commitments. When we compare our views about a range of related cases (using our sensibilities), we are pulled in contrary directions. Indeterminacy is not relativism, however. We are not compelled to relinquish our views about those cases where our commitments are settled. All that we must relinquish, if we go the Humean route, is that we have no way of showing, once and for all, that our views are *the true* views, which everyone must accept on pain of a charge of irrationality.

The fundamental point in all this, to reiterate a point made earlier, is that there are feelings and feelings. The worry about subjectivism and relativism is sharpest if the Humean is interpreted as saying that moral judgments are a matter of "passion" or "sentiment," but this is to understand the Humean in the worst possible light. "We should think in terms of a staircase of practical and emotional ascent," suggests Blackburn.[33] At the bottom are "simple preferences, likes, and dislikes." One step up is "a basic hostility to some kind of action or character or situation: a primitive aversion to it, or a disposition to be disgusted by it, or to hold it in contempt, or to be angered by it, or to avoid it." Beyond this step are more complex, reflective reactions. For example, there are reactions that we come to regard as legitimate, as touching on matters of public concern, and that we would like to see shared by others. Still further up are stances we endorse so strongly that we regard them as compulsory, perhaps even as enforceable. There will be and need be no sharp cut-off point at which a stance becomes a *moral* stance, but generally, "pure preference" is at the bottom of the scale, and it is only in the upper levels that we have "attitudes with all the flavour of ethical commitment." Here, we have stable, considered commitments that are social phenomena in two directions—both in that, for any individual, they will acquired through, confirmed by, and modified by social interactions, and in that the individual will want, to various degrees, to see them taken up in social interactions.

Once we turn to such commitments, we might reasonably expect to find less variety than the subjectivist/relativist worry suggests will arise. Callicott argues that some patterns of emotional reactions are found in all cultures. "The human psychological profile in certain crucial respects is standardized, fixed," writes Callicott. "[A]ll cultures abominate murder, theft, treachery, dishonesty, and other cardinal vices."[34] When moral disagreements arise, asserts Callicott, they stem partly from a variation in the strength and sensitivity of moral sentiment that does not undermine a broad general agreement, partly from different ways of understanding the facts, and partly from disputes about what Callicott calls "proximate values." They are not about the most deeply held values, which Callicott calls "ultimate values." For example, although we may all find some ultimate value in the environment we live in, we may disagree about how to protect it. Some, with one view about the functioning of ecosystems and their importance to the environment, may find some proximate value in top predators—wolves or mountain lions—whereas others, with different views about the ecosystems, regard them merely as vermin.

MORAL ARGUMENT: CONSIDERED JUDGMENTS

The concern about subjectivism and relativism is linked to a second significant concern, which is that the Humean account leaves no room for principled moral argument or moral progress. The emancipation of slaves, the enfranchisement of women, the rejection of racial segregation, and social tolerance of homosexuality all feel like matters of rational progress, not just lateral changes, but if we regard moral reform as consisting strictly of changes in attitudes, then we seem to be forced to abandon any notion of principled argument that could give the experience of moral reform its due. Worse, as I have noted, Hume's own account of debate and deliberation looks rather simplistic, suggesting as it does that moral disagreements collapse quickly into blunt declarations that something seems pleasurable or agreeable, or not.

Fortunately, moral argument comes in a variety of forms, and several of these forms are compatible with Hume's account. The most potent form of moral argument is that which hinges on empirically verifiable facts. It is in this kind of argument that we are most likely to find ourselves cornered and flatly forced to change our stance. In bioethics, the range of factual disputes includes much of what goes on in clinical consulting and aspects of the debates about biotechnology. Disagreements about facts can range from straightforward disputes about the details of the case at hand—who did what to whom, with what likely consequences, and so on—to much larger and more complex debates about world views, scientific theories, theories of human nature, and the like. Nothing in the Humean account requires that this kind of argument be relinquished. Moral judgments are responses to states of affairs in the world, and if we are shown to be wrong about those affairs, then we can be forced to change our moral judgments.

Another frequently effective form of moral argument is that which relies on comparisons to other cases. "How come Rebecca gets big scoops of ice cream and I only get little ones?" Or: "Why is genetic modification of live-stock using gene transfer technology unacceptable if genetic modification of livestock using breeding is acceptable?" We must respond to this kind of argument by giving a reason—by showing that there is a relevant difference between the compared cases—or by changing our judgment about one of the cases. Again, nothing in the Humean account stands in the way of such reasoning. Even in frivolous aesthetic value judgments we can reasonably ask why a person has reached different judgments about two seemingly similar cases. Further up Blackburn's staircase, where more is at stake and where a person making a judgment is not merely expressing his own views but asking others to agree, we can ask for these differences more pointedly.

Finally, we may sometimes have recourse in moral debates to theoretic claims. Even if our working values are a heterogeneous array, we can still look for organizing and ranking principles among them. If we accept that analogical reasoning from one case to another is possible, then we have accepted that abstracting from cases is possible, and we can continue to play that game: we can abstract, then discuss the relationships between abstractions, and so arrive at the generalizations that are rules and princi-ples. These generalizations will be of limited use: if the force of moral judg-ments stems from sentiments, then an abstract observation about those attitudes will usually not cut much ice when we are in the midst of a case. Further, if our moral web is sufficiently complex—if it is a *culture*—then it is unlikely that the generalizations will ever fully capture what we think about the welter of real-life cases. (And, often enough, given competing ways of interpreting and applying the generalizations, they will not get us any closer to a definitive judgment than the welter they are supposed to help organize.) But sometimes they can still be useful, perhaps especially in discussions that occur at some remove from any particular case; they can help us come to better considered positions on difficult classes of cases.

In vitro fertilization (IVF) might initially arouse one's skepticism, for example, on grounds that the production of embryos in test tubes looks too closely akin to manufacture. This is a reaction worth taking seriously, but then worth reassessing—"in the cold hard light of reason," we could almost say. It helps, first, to think about the nature of the relationship between child and parents when the child is created using IVF, about the respects in which creating embryos in test tubes genuinely resembles manufacture, and—if it does not—about the extent to which permitting it is likely to move us toward other methods of creating children that are more like manufacture. These points are examples of arguments about facts. But we must also bear in mind the wide leeway we are already inclined to grant adults who wish to become parents—when, with whom, under what life circumstances, even toward what ends. After thinking about different attitudes we hold that are relevant to the case of IVF, we may decide that our initial skepticism (if we were skeptical) does not carry the day for us. There are other issues at stake that we care about more.

Another general sort of move we can make within the Humean account is to connect moral principles with human wants and needs. Hume holds that human nature leads us to make moral judgments; we might add that human nature also informs those judgments. Mary Midgley develops this notion of argument (although, as noted, without intending it for use in a Humean frame). Midgley holds that morality is rooted in human wants, but she insists that when we turn to human wants, we must talk about human nature rather than merely about what you or I happen to desire just now. The point of morality is to sort out conflicting wants, order them, and get down to fundamentals. The wants we are interested in "are not random impulses. They are articulated, recognizable aspects of life; they are the deepest structural constituents of our characters."[35] (Midgley also holds that wants are best understood not as "passions" but as facts, understanding "facts" as incorporating an evaluative component.) Larry Arnhart goes a similar route, by developing a natural law position that, in explicitly Humean fashion, explains moral imperatives as resting on desire and then turns to Darwin to help identify the "natural desires."[36]

Even if one stops short of a natural law theory, though, plainly, the Humean position can admit that moral judgments are formed, evaluated, and coordinated cognitively. What the Humean position denies is that we can compel a person solely through force of reason to accept a given moral judgment. Furthermore, the Humean position strongly suggests not only that reason is of limited use, but that much effective moral argument will consist in trying to get a person to share one's basic attitudes. We may rely on tone of voice, on stories, on imagery, even on the bonds of friendship, to try to win a person over. But this is just how moral argument actually is. Fortunately, discrepancies in attitudes are rarely chasms; differences are often a matter of emphasis.

Much of the writing of the President's Council that has most frustrated professional philosophers consists of rhetorical moves that seek to persuade rather than to prove. To employ these moves is to admit that one's conclusion cannot be obtained solely by means of inferences. This may be annoying, but so it is with morality.

REPUGNANCE AND REASON

What can be said, then, about a clearly *wrong* moral judgment, such as that white people should be favored over black people in hiring, housing, and other public policy? The worry, of course, is that someone in the grip of the Humean account of moral judgments has nothing much to say: either "Yes, that's right, that's exactly how I feel," or "No, that's not how I feel, although that view is on the same footing as mine."

Somewhere down the line, if the Humean account is right, we may be reduced to saying that this is how we see the matter, but it does not limit us to saying *merely* that about each and every judgment. It can account for the importance that is commonly attached to reevaluating moral views, to asking "Why care about *whites*, particularly? Why should being *white* make a moral difference?"

First, it's important to articulate what it is that people really care about, and the Humean account lets us do this at least as well as any other. Is racism fundamentally a moral stance that could be described as "caring for whites"? Or is it rather more about something else—about caring for the benefits that this unequal social arrangement happens to provide? If racism manifests less as "caring about whites" than as "wanting to keep blacks under," then moral arguments in defense of it are just a veneer to prettify something quite awful. Sometimes, though, even good people are racists. In such cases, there may be a kind of broad factual error—that blacks are lesser people or even that they are not really "people," under some privileged understanding of that term. Also, there are usually multiple values at play: even for racists, "caring about whites" is not the *only* consideration. Even racists can care for *people*. Once the factual error is straightened out, and once some broader principles are identified, the racist can be expected to answer the question, "How is this case different from that?"

Part of what's valuable about moral theorizing—about exploring the extent to which our moral values can be brought under the general heading of "promoting happiness," say—is that it helps us continue to press our questioning, to ask "what's most important here?" Moral judgments are certainly not to be taken at face value and accepted just as they are. Even if they cannot be fully ordered, they are at least to be *coordinated*, as Midgley puts it. The very point of morality, after all, is that it is about what matters *most*: therefore we must (and often will) try to get to the bottom of our values, to articulate them in their most general terms, and also to think about how seemingly competing considerations compare. That we can engage in this kind of coordinating does not mean that we will find some sort of foundation under our values on which the whole system is securely fixed (and which can be deployed to sort out mistakes in the system), but it does mean that we will be able to winnow out some positions.

Such probing will steer us away from regarding skin color as an object of ultimate valuation. It is possibly because moral values cannot be fully ordered, like so many mathematical facts, and are not simply there in the world waiting to be discovered, that racism and sexism can persist even in fundamentally good people. But it is because we can rethink and argue about stances that we can hope eventually to quell racism and sexism.

Will the valuation of nature survive this kind of rethinking and reevaluation? Not necessarily. But it's a good candidate, and it is not surprising that concerns about nature have been growing in significance in a growing range of domains. We cannot (if the argument in this chapter is right) prove that nature should be valued, but we can talk about the valuation of nature in ways that can show why it is, for many people, a compelling if complex ultimate consideration, in somewhat the way that we can talk about reasonableness or happiness in ways that show why those are compelling ultimate considerations. To talk about nature is to consider our "relationship to the cosmos," as Blackburn put in the earlier quotation. To talk about nature is to wrestle with the possibility of our own existence as individuals and as a kingdom of ends, embodied creatures that we are. To talk about nature is to address issues that, for many people, give life meaning, hope, and shape.

The valuation of *specific* "natural" things will almost certainly not always survive rethinking and reevaluation. Stances toward particular natural things may sometimes be abandoned. Later in the book, for example, I will argue that the prospect of synthesizing new kinds of microbes does not pose as great a challenge to the valuation of nature as might be supposed at first blush, when one reads in a newspaper that a scientist has "created a new life-form."

This kind of rethinking can happen in various ways: We might sometimes rethink the degree to which something is natural or the degree to which a given human action interferes with it. That "natural" is both an empirical point and reflects human conventions will make this kind of argument only more complex. There will be trade-offs with other values. An alteration that has a very significant human benefit might be deemed worth it. And there might simply be some flexibility in the idea that we should value nature. It will be useful, for thinking critically about the valuation of nature, to try to articulate the human relationship to nature in a general way, rather than just to list an assortment of things that might be counted as "natural"—species, genomes, human sexual reproduction, pesticide-free farming. We should not assume at the outset, for example, that if it makes sense to speak of the valuation of nature, then we are necessarily affirming some sort of hard and fast general principle—for example, that anything that occurs naturally has value and should, other moral considerations permitting, be left alone.

We should not make this assumption, at least, if we accept the Humean framework. If we assumed instead that value is a real property of things in the world, entirely independent of human observers and merely waiting to be recognized by them, then it would be reasonable to look for firmer rules. (If it is a feature of the world itself that not being a human artifact is connected with value, so that value is to be found wherever nonartifactualness is found, then we would look for very generic rules governing the treatment of all such things.) In the Humean framework, however, it is possible to articulate a principle that is explicitly open-textured, something like this: We should not regard the world as ours to remake however we want. It is commendable sometimes to leave the world alone. Such a principle calls attention to the value attached to nature, but it is articulated not as a point about what a natural state of affairs requires (for example, that if a state of affairs is natural, then it should be left alone) but as a more general point about what kind of human relationship toward nature is deemed desirable (for example, that we ought to try to limit our impact on natural states of affairs).

So understood, the stance we take toward nature will be a little more like the stance we probably take toward promoting happiness. Surely, we agree that people should treat other people in ways that promote their happiness—but we probably do not feel that every interaction ought to promote happiness as much as possible. There is some built-in flexibility in how that principle cashes out in specific actions. Because nature is all-encompassing, because it is strictly impossible to do anything at all without in some way altering nature, if only by breathing and therefore altering atmospheric oxygen and carbon dioxide levels, some specific aspects of nature might be assigned special significance because they signify a larger point about the human relationship to nature: birds of prey might be emblems of the human treatment of nature, or the last remaining example of an ecosystem might have more significance than a similar-sized parcel of land that represents an unthreatened ecosystem. Similarly, the high-altitude, moon-shaped advertising banner might be taken, as Blackburn writes, as "a symptom of a break in the tie between humanity and the cosmos." Likewise, some aspects of human nature might be deemed particularly important.

The plausibility of the Humean account of morality should give us pause about cavalierly dismissing the repugnance Kass finds in biotechnologies that could fundamentally change human life—potentially replacing sexual reproduction, remodeling the parent–child relationship, affecting the child's emerging sense of self, opening the door to further and more significant ways of altering human nature, and changing the way humans see themselves as belonging to the natural world around them. At the same time, if moral judgments issue not just from "feelings" but from considered, stable commitments we have toward our world; stances that reflect the "deepest structural constituents of our characters"; are grounded in basic human wants; and are coordinated, fixed, and developed in human cultures, then we should also not cavalierly accept it. We will not be able to support our positions with arguments that are entirely noncircular: ultimately, our values form a closed system, since they are not grounded on analytic truths or objective features of the universe. But we should still be able to articulate, convey, and defend our views.

We may eventually decide not to do what this sense of repugnance seems to advise. We may find that our initial misgivings diminish as we think more about cloning and how it might be used—with what hopes and goals and to what effect on human lives. We might find that our repugnance dissipates altogether, or we might find that we retain it only about certain uses of cloning—cloning a person without that person's consent, for example, or using cloning to have a child when having a child through the sexual recombination of genes is possible.

In general, we need time to weigh matters. If our moral sentiments have evolved out of and along with the human capacity for cognition and communication, and if they have flowered into cultures that also track their own evolutionary history, then we may struggle to apply them quickly to dramatic changes in human ways of living. We are simply on new ground when we consider what we can do to the "nature" of humans, animals, and the world around us.

NOTES

1. Lee Silver, *Challenging Nature: The Clash between Biotechnology and Spirituality* (New York: HarperCollins, 2006), 297.
2. John Stuart Mill, *Principles of Political Economy*, vol. 2 (London: John Parke, 1848), p. 311. The passage was quoted more completely in Chapter 1.

3. Bernard E. Rollin, *The Frankenstein Syndrome: Ethical and Social Issues in the Genetic Engineering of Animals* (Cambridge, U.K.: Cambridge University Press, 1995).

4. Thomas E. Hill, Jr., "Ideals of Human Excellence and Preserving National Environments," in *Autonomy and Self-Respect* (Cambridge, U.K.: Cambridge University Press, 1991), 104–117.

5. Holmes Rolston, *Environmental Ethics: Duties to and Values in the Natural World* (Philadelphia, Pa.: Temple University Press, 1988).

6. Arne Naess, *Ecology, Community, and Lifestyle: Outline of an Ecosophy* (Cambridge, U.K.: Cambridge University Press, 1989), 28, 51–57.

7. David Hume, *A Treatise of Human Nature*, 2nd ed., ed. L. A. Selby-Bigge (Oxford, U.K.: Oxford University Press, 1978), 275.

8. Ibid., 469.

9. Simon Blackburn, *Ruling Passions: A Theory of Practical Reasoning* (Oxford: Clarendon Press, 1998), vi.

10. David Hume, *Enquiry Concerning Human Understanding*, 3rd ed. (Oxford, U.K.: Oxford University Press, 1975), 169–70.

11. Mary Midgley, *Beast and Man: The Roots of Human Nature* (London, U.K.: Routledge Classics, 2002), 175.

12. For example, John McDowell, "Virtue and Reason," *The Monist* 62 (1979): 331–50; John McDowell, "Non-cognitivism and Rule Following," in *Wittgenstein: To Follow a Rule*, ed. Stephen H. Holtzman and Christopher M. Leich (London: Routledge and Kegan Paul, 1981), 141–61; D. Wiggins, *Needs, Values, Truth: Essays in the Philosophy of Value* (Oxford: Basil Blackwell, 1987); Sabina Lovibond, *Realism and Imagination in Ethics* (Minneapolis, Minn.: University of Minneapolis Press, 1983).

13. Hilde Lindemann, "Autonomy, Beneficence, and Gezelligheid: Lessons in Moral Theory from the Dutch," *Hastings Center Report* 39, no. 5 (2009): 39–45; Hilde Lindemann, "What Child Is This?" *Hastings Center Report* 32, no. 6 (2002): 29–38; James Lindemann Nelson, "'Unlike Calculating Rules?' Clinical Judgment, Formalized Decisionmaking and Wittgenstein," in *Slow Cures and Bad Philosophers: Wittgenstein and Bioethics*, ed. Carl Elliot (Durham, N.C.: Duke University Press, 2001), 48–69; Carl Elliott, *A Philosophical Disease: Bioethics, Culture, and Identity* (New York: Routledge, 1999).

14. J. B. Callicott, "On the Intrinsic Value of Nonhuman Species," in *The Preservation of Species: The Value of Biological Diversity*, ed. B. Norton (Princeton, N.J.: Princeton University Press, 1986), 138–72, 142.

15. Blackburn, *Ruling Passions*, 12.

16. President's Council on Bioethics, *Human Cloning and Human Dignity* (Washington, D.C.: President's Council on Bioethics, 2002), 105.

17. Leon R. Kass, "The Wisdom of Repugnance," *The New Republic* (1997): 17–26, at 20; L. R. Kass, *Life, Liberty, and the Defense of Dignity: The Challenge for Bioethics* (San Francisco, Calif.: Encounter Books, 2002), 150.

18. Chris Mooney, "Irrationalist in Chief," *The American Prospect* 12, no. 7 (2001): 10–12, at 11.

19. Tom L. Beauchamp and James F. Childress, *Principles of Biomedical Ethics*, 4th ed. (New York: Oxford University Press, 1994), 111.

20. Callicott, "On the Intrinsic Value of Nonhuman Species," 156.

21. Ibid., 156.

22. Paul Ehrlich, *Human Natures: Genes, Cultures, and the Human Prospect* (New York: Penguin Books, 2000).

23. S. Blackburn, "Is Objective Moral Justification Possible on a Quasi-Realist Foundation?" *Inquiry* 42 (1999): 213–28.
24. See David Wiggins, "Truth, and Truth as Predicated of Moral Judgments," in *Needs, Values, Truth: Essays in the Philosophy of Value* (Oxford: Basil Blackwell, 1987), 139–84.
25. Bernard Williams, *Ethics and the Limits of Philosophy* (Cambridge, Mass.: Harvard University Press, 1985), 132–48.
26. Eugene Mason, "Holistic Approaches to the Language of Morals," unpublished manuscript.
27. Simon Blackburn, "Securing the Nots: Moral Epistemology for the Quasi-Realist," in *Moral Knowledge? New Readings in Moral Epistemology*, ed. Walter Sinnott-Armstrong and Mark Timmons (New York: Oxford University Press, 1996), 82–100, at 89.
28. Williams, *Ethics and the Limits of Philosophy*, 159.
29. Mary Midgley, *Beast and Man: The Roots of Human Nature* (London, U.K.: Routledge Classics, 2002), 5–6.
30. Blackburn, "Is Objective Moral Justification Possible?" 214.
31. I owe this point to an anonymous reviewer of an earlier version of this chapter.
32. Erik Parens, "Authenticity and Ambivalence: Toward Understanding the Enhancement Debate," *Hastings Center Report* 35, no. 3 (2005): 34–41, at 37.
33. Blackburn, *Ruling Passions*, p. 9. The remaining quotations in this paragraph are from the same source.
34. Callicott, "On the Intrinsic Value of Nonhuman Species," 161.
35. Midgley, *Beast and Man*, 175.
36. Larry Arnhart, *Darwinian Natural Right: The Biological Ethics of Human Nature* (Albany, N.Y.: State University of New York, 1998).

CHAPTER 3

⌁

The "Call of the Wild"

Ideals and Obligations

Some years ago, at a bioethics conference, a physician who had been involved in the treatment of Ashley X, a profoundly cognitively disabled child whose parents had asked doctors to chemically arrest her growth and surgically remove her uterus and breast buds, began a presentation on the intervention by identifying and dismissing what he saw as one of the stupider objections to it. He noted that some people think the interventions are "wrong" because they are "against nature." That was not his view, he said without explanation, and he moved to the next slide. The idea was too ridiculous to discuss.

The guiding intuition in this chapter is that the speaker was right to reject "wrong" but wrong to suggest that the human relationship to nature is not a legitimate topic for moral assessment. But to make that claim is to raise some interesting if perplexing questions about how moral imperatives work. Chapter 2 deployed a broadly Humean account of moral values to argue that nature can be valued, such that the human relationship to nature can be a topic of moral concern. Now some subsidiary questions arise: what *kind of* moral concern would a moral concern about the human relationship to nature be—what kind of moral demands would it support? Suppose that one thinks that leaving a natural place alone can be valuable. What does that valuation call for? Is there a general moral obligation at stake? This chapter aims to explore these questions and to propose (rather than to argue decisively for) an alternative way of thinking about them; it maps out some of the complexities they present, proposes some answers, and argues that those answers have an intuitive plausibility to them.

The question, "What *kind of* moral concern would a moral concern about the human relationship to nature be?" is a bridge of sorts between the second and third general philosophical questions that this book takes up—the questions, that is, of whether nature can be a legitimate subject of moral concern and whether attitudes toward nature can be taken up into public discourse and public policy making. Part of the opposition to the philosophical claim that nature can be a legitimate subject of moral concern is that it appears to lead to some awkward-sounding *moral* claims, such as that doing something "against nature" is *wrong*. Getting clearer on what kind of assessments a moral concern about nature supports—clearing away the awkwardness, if we can—would provide further support to the idea that nature can be a legitimate topic of moral concern. (And if the helpful clarification makes use of and depends on the Humean account, then it provides support for that account by showing how the account allows us to make more overall sense of the moral landscape.) At the same time, getting clearer on this question might also shed light on the role that concerns about nature play or should play, not only in an individual's life, but also in interpersonal moral assessments, in public discourse, and in a society's drafting of public policy. If a person cares morally about the human relationship to nature, would that person also feel—ought that person feel—that everyone else should care about nature, too? Might one conclude, for example, that a given human intervention into nature is *wrong*, that somebody who acts that way is *guilty* of doing something wrong, and therefore perhaps that the action should be forbidden by law?

DUTIES TOWARD NATURE

Once again, environmental ethics provides a useful way of opening up the problem. Environmental ethics has repeatedly explored the nature of the moral relationship to nature. One colorful exploration that is consistent with the approach to concepts and values offered in this book, and that expressly seeks to consider how the relationship to nature fits alongside other moral concerns, is that offered by Mary Midgley in a paper titled "Duties Concerning Islands." Midgley starts by proposing a possible entry in the journal kept by Robinson Crusoe:

19 Sept. 1685. This day I set aside to devastate my island. My pinnance being now ready on the shore, and all things prepared for my departure, Friday's people also

expecting me, and the wind blowing fresh away from my little harbour, I had a mind to
see how all would burn. So then, setting sparks and powder craftily among certain dry
spinneys which I had chosen, I soon had it ablaze, nor was there left, by the next dawn,
any green stick among the ruins.[1]

"Work on the style how you will," declares Midgley, the entry is not cred-
ible. "Crusoe was not the most scrupulous of men, but he would have felt
an invincible objection to this senseless destruction. So would the rest of
us." Midgley's view appears to be (although I shall note a complication later
on) that human intervention into a natural state of affairs can be flatly
wrong. The human relationship to the environment stands alongside other
moral concerns. Midgley does not expressly consider how duties concerning islands might enter into public policy making concerning islands, but
by characterizing the moral attitude with the language of duty, she has laid
some of the groundwork for concluding that certain ways of treating the
natural world could be legally forbidden.

Midgley's strong stance is the going position in environmental ethics.
Aldo Leopold helped launched the field by describing the moral value in relatively strong terms, and environmental ethics has mostly followed suit. "A
thing is right when it tends to preserve the integrity, stability, and beauty
of the biotic community," Leopold declared. "It is wrong when it tends otherwise."[2] Leopold called this view the "land ethic," and he described it as
a simple extension of the notion of moral obligation, which was initially
applied to relations between individuals and later broadened to address the
relations between individuals and society. "The land ethic simply enlarges
the boundaries of the community to include soils, waters, plants, and animals, or collectively: the land."[3]

Midgley's argument for the strong position consists in part of clearing
away philosophical objections to it—a task that she undertakes primarily by
arguing that the range of moral duties is not limited by the idea that a duty
involves a corresponding right and therefore a sentient rights-holder—and
also, in part, of appealing to the felt force of the moral concern—which
she accomplishes in good measure by laying out the example just given.
I return to the phenomenological question later.

First, though, I want to note that many others in environmental ethics
have tried to do rather more than appeal to the felt force; they have thought
that the force of the moral concern about the human relationship to nature
requires a special philosophical explanation. This might be explained, for
example, by holding that duties toward the environment flow from divine
directives—that some ways of treating nature are, as it were, abomina-
tions unto nature. The typical move in environmental ethics, however, is to

establish that the distinction between humans and nature is also a meta-physical distinction, not just what Kate Soper calls a "lay" distinction—a distinction that makes empirical claims, yet in a way that is framed by convention—and the moral urgency of the relationship to nature stems from this metaphysical distinction.[4]

For example, the environmental ethicist Eric Katz, who described the theme of a collection of his essays as the view "that humanity has moral obligations to the natural world, similar to the obligations that exist from one human being to another, to preserve its integrity, identity, and free development," argues that the threat that humans pose to nature is not just about environmental degradation and the extinction of species; in Katz's view, it is also about control.[5] A forest that has come under human control—a managed forest—might not show any environmental damage and might provide a home to all of the species that could be found on the same site in an unmanaged forest, but it is still a loss to the natural world. It is a loss of nature's autonomy. Nature, understood here as a realm entirely free of human influence, is replaced by artifact, which cannot be understood and does not exist except on the strength of human intentions. (Katz describes artifacts as having an ontological dependence on intentions.) The moral question, then, is about human domination of nature, the imperialistic exercise of power over nature.

This kind of formulation lends itself to a strong stance. "Need we ask why domination is a moral issue?" writes Katz.[6] To speak of *domination* is to simply declare that evil is at stake. Katz concludes that there are "obligations on the part of humanity for the preservation and protection of the natural world. This is the *call of the wild*—the moral claim of the natural world."

Making sense of the idea that human alteration of nature amounts to infringement on nature's autonomy runs into various problems, of course. One set of problems is that, since Katz defines "natural" as flatly inconsistent with the presence of human intentionality, he is committed to an absolutist view of how the concept of nature works. I argued in Chapter 1 that an absolutist understanding is not necessary, and in Chapter 5 I will articulate a nonabsolutist understanding of nature more thoroughly in the context of environmentalist concerns. Here, I want only to point out that the reason for developing a nonabsolutist position on "nature" is that the absolutist understanding is so hard to defend. First, it becomes much more awkward to sort out the many things that seem to fall somewhere in the middle. Katz tries to avoid this kind of problem by suggesting that whereas "nature" is defined as the absolute absence of human intentionality, actual physical things partake of the *property* of naturalness to varying degrees and that we can speak of those things as being natural to degrees even while the property of nature is defined as absolutely free of human intentionality. But this may still lead to positions that some find counterintuitive. By this definition, for example, an organic garden is as unnatural as a gravel parking lot, since the varieties of plants in it, their arrangement on the ground, and probably the soil itself reflect human intentionality. Sites that have been damaged but do not reflect thorough human design—an abandoned dump left undisturbed or a forest taken over by an invasive species—would have to be considered more natural than a site that has been carefully "returned to nature," since to plant anything on a dump would be to preserve its artifactual character.

Katz's strong understanding of moral obligations to nature also lead him into some metaphysical positions that will be challenging to defend—a point that I table for now, since I take it up in depth in Chapter 5. Finally, there are problems with applying the notions of domination and autonomy to nature in the way Katz does. One problem is that there are disanalogies between human "domination" of other humans and human domination of nature. Nature is not autonomous in the same way as human beings. We can recognize some of these disanalogies without giving up on saying that humans are dominating nature, but, at some point, we lose some of the moral overtones. There would be some sense in describing a carpenter as dominating a piece of wood, but there is no moral force to that kind of domination. Another problem is that, strictly speaking, given Katz's account of nature and artifact, nature *cannot* be controlled by humans; it can only be squeezed out. When humans assert control over a natural thing, it simply ceases to be natural. Nature can cede ground to humans, but it cannot be *dominated* by humans.

THE IDEAL OF NATURE

These problems arise out of an effort to make the "call of the wild" a morally strong command. The point of Katz's account of "nature"—of what distinguishes "natural" from "artificial"—is to show that the moral commands nature issues are clear and are rooted in something having to do with nature itself, rather than in human culture. If the account succeeded, it would establish that the moral requirements of the human relationship to nature are strong and real—a feature of the universe as it is, in no sense a cultural construction. In short, protecting the environment is a universal moral obligation, binding on all people. In fact, however, there is good reason to think that the "call of the wild" is considerably more complicated.

Consider an example offered by the Kantian moral philosopher Thomas Hill, who, like Midgley, expressly seeks to consider how the relationship to nature fits alongside other moral concerns:

> A wealthy eccentric bought a house in a neighborhood I know. The house was surrounded by a beautiful display of grass, plants, and flowers, and it was shaded by a huge avocado tree. But the grass required cutting, the flowers needed tending, and the man wanted more sun. So he cut the whole lot down and covered the yard with asphalt. After all it was his property and he was not fond of plants.[7]

Now what is the right reaction to such behavior? To someone who shares a concern for nature, it seems unattractive, and one could add details to the story that make the landowner's behavior downright despicable (perhaps the man knows the loss will be mourned by someone he knows, and he relishes that thought). But as described here, is it wrong?

Hill's goal is to account for environmentalist moral concerns within a Kantian framework and without relying on what he sees as dubious claims about the moral status of nature—such as that plants have rights, that it is God's will we care for nature, or that nature possesses intrinsic value. (I argued in Chapter 2 that the idea of finding intrinsic value in nature is not dubious within a Humean framework, but Hill has in mind a non-Humean claim that the value is genuinely there in the world, only waiting to be discovered.) Hill suggests that even if nature does not itself have value, virtuous people might *tend to value nature*. Caring for nonsentient nature is connected with other virtues or excellences, such as an aesthetic sense and gratitude, and indifference to nature is connected with human vices, such as ignorance and self-importance.[8] The connection Hill envisions is not one of logical necessity: caring for nonsentient nature does not *necessarily* reflect virtue, and lack of caring does not necessarily reflect vice. Nonetheless, argues Hill, it tends to be the case that virtuous people have an attitude of respect and appreciation for nature.

This account will seem hopelessly underpowered to someone like Katz. Valuing nature only *may* reflect a kind of humility, a recognition and even appreciation of the fact that one is part of a larger whole—the natural order to which we all belong. It need not. "Even if experiencing nature promotes humility..., there may be other ways people can develop such humility in a world of concrete, glass, and plastic."[9] And Hill certainly supposes that nature does not actually have moral value. Here, concern for nature is made into an accidental by-product of virtue, merely derivative from true moral concerns, which have to do with humans; for Katz and many other environmentalists, nature is itself a subject of moral concern, even if that concern might be secondary to concern for fellow human beings.

Hill himself seems dissatisfied with what he says about the importance of moral concern for nature. In a later paper, he searches for a reason that a virtuous person might indeed be *required* to value nature. The core idea is that a virtuous person would have to be ready to appreciate the good in all sorts of things, the natural world among them. "There seems to be something important missing in those who persistently ignore, cynically dismiss, or remain coldly indifferent to the vast range of things that are sources of joy, inspiration and value for others, and potentially for themselves."[10] A person who possesses this general virtue will have the specific virtue of appreciating the value of nature, Hill argues, at least if we can sensibly say that there really is value there to be found, independent of claims about human welfare and rights and without wandering into the metaphysical thickets we would find ourselves in if we began speaking of intrinsic values as "independently existing natural (or 'non-natural') properties of things."[11] Hill then argues that we can sensibly ascribe value to nature—not merely that it is valued—if by "valuable in itself" we mean only "that its being valued is not (or need not be) simply the result of mistakes of various kinds—for example, failure to understand it, confusion, bad reasoning, judgment skewed by irrelevant biases, and so on."[12] If people valued a thing because they had been indoctrinated, for example, and we thought they would recant if they gave the matter a careful, critical analysis and were freed of indoctrination, then we would not say that the thing was "valuable in itself." That those people valued it was just a quirk of circumstance. Hill assumes that nature will make the cut and count as "valuable in itself" in this sense.

Hill's revisions will still look weak to Katz. The account of what it means for something to be "valuable in itself" comes up well shy of establishing that the thing is making normative demands on one; to say that people are not being silly when they find value in something is not yet to say that everybody ought to value that thing. Nor does the general virtue of being *ready* to appreciate the good in all sorts of things impel one to appreciate the good in any *one* thing. Many millions of people seem to find stock car racing a source of joy, inspiration, and value, but that does not mean that every virtuous person should find pleasure in it.

Perhaps Hill simply ought to give up trying to satisfy Katz's normative standards and hold that what his account seeks to establish is that the valuation of nature is not a mistake, but not that it *is* a mistake to *fail* to share that valuation. In other words, perhaps the goal need not be showing that concern for nature is obligatory, in the usual sense of obligation: concern for nature cannot be expected of any good person. Some actions or stances are inconsistent with being a good person, but maybe one can be a good person and still fail to value nature in itself. There might be an element of optionality in this stance and in actions reflecting it.

Most vegetarians I know (although not all I know *of*) think of vegetarianism this way: they have reached a moral decision not to eat meat, they applaud others who come to that view, they might try to persuade others to come to that view, but they would probably stop short of saying that eating meat is flatly wrong or that people who eat meat are bad people. They will skirt somewhere just outside this view; they will say that they have strong opinions about eating meat, that they now find the thought of eating meat revolting, and that they are delighted when people around them turn out to share their views, but they will nonetheless leave leeway for views that depart from theirs. In short, vegetarianism is a position to which they are personally deeply committed and which they would like to see in others, but carnivorousness does not (in their view) warrant social condemnation. The science journalist Michael Pollan has evoked, in an interview, a similar position about growing and preparing vegetables: "The longer I'm at it, the more I'm convinced that gardening and cooking are really important activities, both at a practical level and at a spiritual or philosophical level. Both are ways to reconnect with the earth, with all the processes that keep us alive."[13] Maybe—and Pollan is within his rights in recommending the practice to others by calling it "really important"—but he is also right to stop there and not add that everyone *must* do it. Finally, perhaps something similar might be said about some of the moral projects around which people organize their lives—monkish contemplation or political activism, commitment to a family or to a community: these are really important to individuals, and people living in these ways could well want to draw in others, but, surely, it is not the case that everyone must do it.

At the heart of the moral life is a large swath in which we speak of behavior as being right or correct, as a matter of obligation or duty. Somewhere nearby are various kinds of behavior that can be commendable without being obligatory, for various reasons. One possible reason is that they are supererogatory in a traditional sense. Some actions might be simply above and beyond the call of duty. They might be supreme acts of charity or self-abnegating assistance to others, for example. These acts are widely recognized as good—indeed, as very good—but not as required. Another reason actions might be nonobligatory is that they do not *rise to* the level of duty. Small acts of kindness fall into this category. Actions in this category can also be called supererogatory, if by that we do not mean specifically what goes above and beyond duty, but more generally that which is outside the reach of duty. The visual metaphor for both these types of nonobligatory behavior is that of a vertical scale with a kind of horizontal line across the middle marking behavior that is required by duty. The classic understanding of supererogatory action is that of actions above the line; under a broader understanding sometimes employed, supererogatory action is either above or below the line.

Perhaps there are still other aspects of the supererogatory. Could a moral standard be recognizable to a person feeling it as having ordinary strength—being neither above nor below what duty requires—yet still not be seen as a matter of general obligation, incumbent on all people? If so, then a vertical scale might be insufficient to capture the full variety of moral standards. Perhaps we need another visual metaphor to depict this aspect of the nonobligatory—a metaphor like a web. Moral commitments that can generate general obligations would be near the center; commitments that are not accepted as generating such claims would be further out. Even for the central moral commitments, a possible course of action might be nonobligatory because it is supererogatory in one of the two senses mentioned earlier, but the noncentral commitments would be nonobligatory for other kinds of reasons. To some extent, people may simply stake out different patterns—different sets of nodes, as it were—within the overall web.

One reason—or set of reasons—that we might offer to explain why some moral commitments are not central and are nonobligatory is the lack of consensus within the moral community. There can be disagreement about facts (for example, about the degree of similarity between animals' capacities for experiencing pain and suffering and those of humans, thus generating disagreement about how far to go in extending to animals our standards for the treatment of humans), about values (for example, about the implications of humility or about the moral weight that should be attached to it), or about metaphysics (for example, about whether one has moral obligations to God). It is a recurring feature of moral deliberation that we have different but overlapping moral world views, that we recognize this plurality of views, and that we are constantly communicating and negotiating with others about our differences and commonalities. Indeed, this may be more than just a neutral fact about the moral life; it may have both undesirable and desirable consequences, as it both leads to moral disputes and makes for cultural variety and richness. But where we recognize that reasonable people can have different views on some question of value, we have reason not to hold that everyone must endorse the same standards of character and conduct, even though those standards may be very important to those of us who hold them.

The moral life is also conditioned by a more *individual* variability. Through some combination of innate disposition and environmental factors, some people are more motivated by, and may be better at, some aspects of the moral life than others. Their lives coalesce around certain sets of nodes within the web. Some people are activists, some nurturers; some are abstract and rational, some concrete and warm; some tend toward going their own way, some toward building community; some tend toward privacy, others toward candor; and so on. Differences in how much people *care* about a value will sometimes take the form of straightforward disagreements about it. But these differences cannot always be articulated that way. Consider how somebody who, motivated by injustices in her community, seeks political office and rises to an important position is different from somebody who, moved by the same injustices, enthusiastically votes for her but is otherwise not politically active. The politician draws a salary; even if she is doing great work, we would probably not describe her as *saintly*— that is, as engaged in work that is supererogatory in the usual sense of going above and beyond what duty requires. Nor is her work well described as being *less* than what duty requires; the values are very important, and let us suppose that what she is accomplishing as she works toward them is significant. Rather, she is simply pulled especially strongly toward some kinds of moral values and toward work that honors those values, to the point that we might say she has a particular understanding of the kind of life she wants to lead. (Suppose, too, that the politician pays a kind of moral price for leading this life; perhaps she does not spend as much time or energy in her relationships with her husband or children as she wishes—she is not the kind of spouse or parent that she most admires. The moral cost might not be so great that we would say she has chosen her life poorly, but it would give additional reason to say that she has not achieved sainthood by becoming a politician.) Again, although perhaps many or all of these individual tendencies can involve moral problems of one sort or another when they take extreme forms, this variability, like the first, might nonetheless also be an attractive feature of the moral life. It, too, is part and parcel of the diversity and richness of human experience. This variability, too, would lead us to say that a behavior specified by a moral standard is, although perhaps very important to those who hold it, not generally obligatory.

The cultural and individual variability of the moral life is unsurprising if we think of the moral life not just as something individuals do, but rather as something people do socially. We do not, cannot, examine how our lives square with our values simply by thinking it over in private very carefully. Because values are fuzzy, their "implications" unclear, and the process of moral deliberation so very unlike an algorithm, we set about trying to figure out what our values require in good measure just by seeing what they are generally held to require. Moreover, we do not simply consider how well we are living by our values; we must also constantly examine our values, and that is in good measure a social process. We must constantly assess and negotiate our differences with others. The metaphor of the web easily lends itself to this fact; the web maps onto the use of a web as a visual metaphor for a conceptual scheme. By contrast, the strictly vertical representation of the supererogatory, in which the nonobligatory is either above or below the line marking duty, is not connected to that kind of variability and may even lend itself to the idea that there is a common set of moral standards that bear equally on all people.

Yet neither social disagreement nor individual variation in moral psychology fully explains why some standards are closer to the supererogatory than to the obligatory. Some social disagreements are precisely about where an "ought" lies, and some individual variations just need correcting. Might there be a final and more brute sense in which a moral standard does not involve obligation? Namely, that the individuals who recognize it should see it as bearing on themselves rather than on all people? Such a standard would be a goal endorsed by individuals for orienting their lives rather than a goal enforced by society. We might call such a standard a personal "ideal" rather than a social obligation, understanding an ideal as being simply what we have been delineating but without adverting to social consensus or individual make-up to explain it: a standard of character or conduct that one at least aspires to achieve or live by oneself and perhaps even feels morally compelled toward, but that one does not think is morally compelled of every good person. Someone who lives a contemplative life, for example, might feel that the life of contemplation is morally important for her, but not necessarily required of everybody else, and she might not feel that she can explain why she applies that standard especially to herself merely by appealing to lack of social consensus or her own unique attributes. Can there be such a moral standard? Under traditional philosophical positions, in which moral values are oriented toward larger ends such as happiness or the dignity of a rational will, perhaps not; but if we accept the Humean account, then there is no obvious structural impediment to recognizing them. If moral standards are projections on the world of human attitudinal stances, then why not allow that, within the complex social web of moral standards, there arise some that are endorsed by individuals specially to guide their own lives?

It seems to me that all of these considerations about the supererogatory are plausible and that it is a virtue of the Humean account that it can accommodate them. (Perhaps, if we accept a broadly Humean account, we would even expect to find that some moral standards meet the description here, for if moral positions are articulated in "thick," socially complex terms and encompass a range of commitment—not just one but several of the topmost steps on Blackburn's "staircase"[14]—then perhaps the account here fills a gap.) It also seems to me that all of these considerations apply in some measure to what Katz labels "the call of the wild." It is indeed a *call*, we might say—a *calling*—more than a *command*. Working assiduously to protect bits and pieces of nature is above and beyond what can be expected of any individual, and the value of protecting nature may simply not be as strong as other, more central values (it may be a step lower on the staircase). Also, both cultural and individual variability are characteristic of moral concern about nature. Not everyone even recognizes it. The call of the wild can be motivated by a strong sense of the interconnectedness of all living things, for instance, but this sense, much though there might be to recommend it, need not be part of the worldview of all morally sensible people. Some are struck much more by the competition among things and the urge each living thing feels to advance its own cause. Some are impressed less that we should value the world as we find it than that we should strive to master the world and build a better life on it. And, setting aside underlying disagreements, the call of the wild is simply not as loud and plaintive to some people as it is to others. Just as some people may care primarily about rectifying social problems, or about interacting with others in a warm and friendly way, or about fostering individuality and self-sufficiency, one may be moved more or less by the call of the wild.

MORAL SERIOUSNESS

The idea that some value judgments are nonobligatory for the just-stated reasons is a contentious claim, and I do not suppose I have accomplished a full defense of it here. I hope only to have set out the general shape of the idea, in hopes of making it appear intuitively plausible. But it might be possible to incorporate some of the moral complexity I am calling for—the variation in whether and how we expect other sensible people to agree with our moral stances—without relinquishing the language of "obligation."

Undoubtedly, one thing that's attractive about the view that the call of the wild expresses an obligation is that it captures this feeling that the call is loud and plaintive and that the moral response to it feels significant and serious—an important theme in a moral life. Understanding it as an obligation, on all fours with other moral obligations, would be one way of giving it significance and seriousness, and it would be a simpler, more straightforward route than trying to allow that a value stance might be very important to the individuals sharing it yet not be a stance that *everyone* must share.

Midgley's depiction of Robinson Crusoe as a pyromaniac delighting in the wanton destruction of nature supports the direct route: readers will agree, Midgley supposes, that Crusoe violates a moral duty when he destroys every green stick on his island. As the argument develops, however, Midgley makes a move similar, in ways, to the one I have roughly blocked out: she points out that the moral commitment to nature differs from some other moral commitments in that it does not involve the framework of contract—that is, of a binding agreement between rational adults. To speak of what is binding is, in Midgley's argument, to speak of what is socially enforceable, either legally or through other mechanisms. Thus, Midgley is close to accomplishing the same thing, but by using different conceptual tools: she, too, moves the moral commitment to nature outside the range of what is socially enforceable while retaining the language of duty and obligation. She simply complicates those concepts by showing that they can be dissociated from the framework of a contract: "Duties need *not* be quasi-contractual relations between symmetrical pairs of rational human agents. There are all kinds of other obligations holding between asymmetrical pairs, or involving ... no outside beings at all."[15]

Midgley's position may still look different, though: her reason for retaining "duty" and "obligation" is to preserve the seriousness and commitment that such language conveys and that might seem lacking in the account given earlier of the supererogatory: "To speak of duties *to* things in the inanimate and comprehensive sectors ... expresses merely that there are suitable and unsuitable ways of behaving in given situations."[16] If the moral stance toward nature is not understood as a duty, then it looks to be "a matter of taste, style or feeling, of aesthetic sensibility, of habit and nostalgia, of etiquette and local custom, [and not] something which demands our attention whether we like it or not."[17]

If the point of the language of obligation is only to maintain moral seriousness, perhaps we can indeed keep that language after all, merely adding that we are using it a little differently from how some others use it. Certainly, the stance toward nature feels like obligation from within; it is felt as *demanding our attention*, even as *binding*. The key point is that we incorporate enough complexity in our understanding of moral values to allow that social enforceability is not always part of the story—or, at least, that our understanding of social enforceability must itself have various renderings. For Midgley, the words "rights" and "duties" "do indeed have narrow senses approximating to the legal, but they also have much wider ones in which they cover the whole moral sphere."[18] If duty equals obligation, as Midgley supposes, then it is also part of her thesis that the language of obligation likewise has a narrow sense approximating to the legal and a wider sense covering the whole moral sphere. The narrow sense approximating to the legal is that in which social enforceability comes into play. In the broader sense, social enforceability is either not permissible or must be understood as amounting to something softer, slower, and less sure: rather than demand right action, we sometimes only encourage it; rather than expect that a sensible person will do what is right, we sometimes merely seek to inculcate in a sensible person the value stance we deem right.

Of course, there will be many cases in which the moral commitment concerning one's relationship to nature is indeed a matter of obligation, even in the narrower sense. We are narrowly obligated to abide by laws enacted to protect the environment. We are narrowly obligated to honor contracts and promises we have made that commit us to environmental action. We are narrowly obligated to avoid causing environmental damage that we know will endanger the public health. But the source of the obligation in these cases is our relationship with other people, not our relationship to the environment. In these cases, there is, after all, an element of contract, explicit to varying degrees: we are obligated to keep agreements, to follow legitimately enacted laws, and not to harm others.

Perhaps, too, we are also obligated to show some level of respect for other people's deeply held values, even if we do not share them ourselves. One way to do that is to carve out some public space in which those others can uphold their values and, if possible, even to treat that space as itself having value. If my neighbor tells me tearfully that his dog has died and asks me to hold his hands while he prays for the dog's soul, I am probably obligated to observe silence even if I find his thoughts about the dog's soul amusing. Here, it is respect for my neighbor that is the source of my obligation. Similarly, if my neighbor, who is an avid birder, tells me of a rare bird that has stopped over in our vicinity while migrating, and I then spot my cat (also an avid birder, albeit in a different way) stalking that very bird in my backyard, respect for my neighbor's values probably gives me an obligation to shoo my cat away, even if I have no interest in birds.

When obligation arises in these indirect ways, the motivation we expect of the person who is under the obligation seems to shift accordingly: we do not require that people *feel the need* to preserve wetlands or species. We require only that they do it. The motivating factor is one's commitment to contracts, law, or respect for others.

Finally, perhaps something very close to obligation can creep back into the picture even if we set aside cases in which contractual or contract-like relations with other people provide obligation indirectly. Midgley's example of Crusoe burning his island is specially chosen to peel away any element of contract; until Crusoe is rescued, there is nobody else around. It is also specially chosen to be highly destructive, as the destructiveness generates a sense of umbrage and helps underwrite the feeling that a full-fledged *ought* is at stake: people ought not demolish tropical islands. Hill's example, of a neighbor replacing the plantings on his yard with pavement, is less dramatic; it is less likely that rare species, unique habitats, or special ecosystems have been permanently lost.

In short, cases involving the destruction of nature come in a range of flavors. They may involve the destruction of specific plants or animals, of members of a rare species, of an entire species, of an interrelating set of plants and animals, of a rare ecosystem, or of a notable geological formation. They may also involve the introduction of new species or other changes to the existing balance. There are also cases in which a concern about the human relationship to nature would be intermixed with additional moral considerations, as when the destruction includes air pollution, water pollution, or a significant contribution to global warming. If our array of examples is wide enough, many of them will seem appropriate for an ever more strenuous and serious attempt to inculcate the "right" views in a person—a kind of pressure that can gradually rise to something that will be indistinguishable from "social enforcement." Many other cases, though, will not be occasions for argument.

Perhaps we have a "moral obligation" not to ruin tropical islands for sport. But this would be a very special case, featuring spectacular and permanent destruction that is offset only by the fleeting delight in witnessing the conflagration. Most cases would be more like Hill's. Given the overall range of cases, what does it mean to say that obligation pertains in cases involving particularly great destruction? Is the point that we can still sometimes have a duty toward nature or that we ought not engage in wanton destruction of things that matter deeply to many people? Examples involving the destruction of famous works of art or important archeological artifacts would arouse similar sentiments. Either way, most cases involving the human relationship to nature can still fit into the paradigm of a moral ideal, in which the moral compulsion is not socially enforceable. We are simply left recognizing that the boundary between ideal and obligation (understood outside the frame of contract) is not distinct.

In considering the scenario that opened this chapter, I would not describe the interventions performed on Ashley's body as being "against nature" and therefore *wrong*. Part of the problem is with the account of nature that is implicit in the phrase "against nature"—a point that I take up in Chapter 8. Another part of the problem with that judgment is that, insofar as we are talking about the human relationship to nature, "wrong" strikes me as the wrong *kind of judgment*. I would be disinclined (I think) to make the bodily changes that Ashley's parents sought, but I shy away from regarding Ashley's parents' decision as a moral *mistake*. Additionally, my own experience as a parent is so different from that of Ashley's parents that I cannot really get at some of the facts of the case—I do not really know what they are going through—and so I cannot quite say what I would do if she were my daughter. My guess is that I would not have wanted those interventions. But I do not condemn her parents for seeking them.

NOTES

1. Mary Midgley, "Duties Concerning Islands," in *Environmental Ethics*, ed. Robert Elliot (Oxford: Oxford University Press, 1995), 89–103, at 89.
2. Aldo Leopold, *A Sand County Almanac, And Sketches Here and There* (Oxford: Oxford University Press, 1949), 224–25.
3. Ibid., 204.
4. Kate Soper, *What Is Nature? Culture, Politics, and the Non-Human* (Oxford, U.K.: Blackwell, 1995), 156.
5. Eric Katz, *Nature as Subject: Human Obligation and Natural Community* (Lanham, Md.: Rowman & Littlefield Publishers, 1997), xxv.
6. Katz, Nature as Subject, 117.
7. Thomas E. Hill, Jr., "Ideals of Human Excellence and Preserving Natural Environments," in *Autonomy and Self-Respect* (Cambridge: Cambridge University Press, 1991), 104–17.
8. Hill, "Ideals of Human Excellence and Preserving Natural Environments," 109.
9. Ibid., 113.
10. Thomas Hill, "Finding Value in Nature," *Environmental Ethics* 15, no. 3, (2006), 331–41, at 334.
11. Ibid., 335.
12. Ibid., 336.
13. Therese Ciesinski, "A Conversation with Michael Pollan," *Organic Gardening*, November 26, 2010, http://www.organicgardening.com/living/conversation-michael-pollan.
14. Simon Blackburn, *Ruling Passions: A Theory of Practical Reasoning* (Oxford: Clarendon Press, 1998), 9. Blackburn's account is discussed in Chapter 2.
15. Midgley, "Duties Concerning Islands," 101.
16. Ibid., 101.
17. Ibid., 94.
18. Ibid., 94.

CHAPTER 4

Space for Nature

Intrinsic Moral Values in Public Policy

It is easy to tacitly assume that the moral judgments we reach about the human relationship to nature should be closely mirrored by public policy. This assumption came right to the surface when Mark McGwire, Sammy Sosa, Rafael Palmeiro, Jose Canseco, and Curt Schilling sat down before the US House of Representatives Committee on Oversight and Government Reform in March 2005 to discuss steroid use in baseball. Senator Jim Bunning of Kentucky, a Hall of Fame pitcher in the 1950s and '60s who also testified before the committee, put his view this way: "Since the beginning of this scandal, I have said that baseball should get the chance to clean up its own mess, and government should stay out of the way. With the new steroid testing policy, it looks like baseball has taken a first baby step toward restoring honesty to the game. But if they backslide, or don't follow through, then the owners and players need to know that we can and will act."[1] The hearings touched on an assortment of possible reasons for taking action, and the human relationship to nature was among them. Again, Bunning: "When I played with Henry Aaron, Willie Mays and Ted Williams, they didn't put on 40 pounds ... and they didn't hit more home runs in their late thirties as they did in their late twenties. What's happening in baseball is not natural, and it's not right." Bunning thought the government should be ready to weigh in: "If baseball fails to fix this scandal, there are a lot of things we can do to get their attention—by amending the labor laws, repealing the outdated antitrust exemption that baseball alone enjoys, and shining the spotlight of public scrutiny."

Congress did not follow up on Bunning's threat; Major League Baseball still controls steroid policy—although, in a sense, merely holding hearings itself constituted public policy on the issue, insofar as it underscored the seriousness of the issue (shining the light of public scrutiny), gave some guidance as to what actions the league should take, and forced the league into taking action by means of sheer public pressure. On some other topics, government has been more direct. The Endangered Species Act is grounded on the view that humans should try to avoid driving other species into extinction, and marriage laws in most states have long been written so as to enforce a traditional view of natural human sexuality (although, I am pleased to say, this policy is now changing almost faster than I can write).

Much scholarly work on the human relationship to nature seems to accept that if human enhancement is intrinsically wrong, then we ought to do something to stop it. In general, however, whether a moral concern should lead to policy is frequently a complicated business; it may not, and if it should, *how* it affects policy may be complicated. Cruelty is very wrong, and yet many cases of cruelty lie outside the law's reach. Lying is frequently wrong, but the state enforces honesty only in a subset of cases—when testifying in court, for example. Kindness is widely accepted as desirable, yet the government does little to promote it. Given all of the complications of moral ideals described in the previous chapter, how they intersect with policy seems likely to be even more complicated.

In short, even if we conclude that the concept of nature is coherent and that moral views about the human relationship to nature can be legitimate, still we are left with a third general question: how should these concerns be taken up into public discourse and public policy making? By and large, a quick survey of prominent positions in political philosophy—which I attempt in the first portions of this chapter—suggests that, although morality and policy are connected, we should guard against overreaching and should, on many moral matters, strive for middling positions. Once we are beyond certain core moral issues that are crucial to the functioning of the state, we should aim for policy that seeks to carve out a space in which people can live by their views but that does not either impose or exclude any of them. These regions include rich conceptions of what makes for a good life and claims about the human relationship to nature. In the latter part of this chapter, however, I argue that "carving out a space" will tend to push government toward more active support than one might guess— toward modest engagement with citizens' rich moral conceptions rather than toward what we might think of as a "hands-off" stance. "Carving out a space" will amount to a constantly contested set of exchanges from issue to issue; since positive support for one value will sometimes impede a competing value, the exercise of government power to carve out space will be a difficult and ever-changing task. Thus, the question of how moral views about nature may legitimately figure in public policy making will need to be taken up case by case; the goal in this chapter is to secure that conclusion and lay some groundwork for the case-by-case analysis.

ALTERNATIVE POLITICAL PHILOSOPHIES

Some environmental philosophers simply reject the going views in political philosophy. For them, these views are implausibly anthropocentric.[2] They think that nature should be included in the range of things that are part of the moral community—that as the jurisprudential scholar Christopher Stone once suggested, trees should have standing, too[3]—not just that nature is a subject about which humans have strongly felt but divergent moral opinions. For Stone, including nature within the political community is the force of Aldo Leopold's "land ethic," which included the environment in the moral community. The obvious immediate reaction, as Stone notes, is that trees and mountains are not people; the political community is a community of people, and trees and mountains are excluded from the community by definition. But this objection does not go through quite as straightforwardly as one might think; Stone points out that what counts as a "person" is largely a legal fiction; in the case of persons who are not rational adult human beings, we allow that their rights may be represented by other agents.

The more important issues have to do with justice. If we do not restrict the political community to *rational agents*, then the current basic principles of political legitimacy become unworkable. John Rawls, one of the leading lights in twentieth-century political philosophy, asserts that the liberal state adheres to a "principle of legitimacy": "Our exercise of political power is proper and hence justifiable only when it is exercised in accordance with a constitution the essentials of which all citizens may reasonably be expected to endorse in light of principles and ideals acceptable to them as reasonable and rational."[4] The principle supposes that members of the political community have moral powers that allow them to judge things reasonable and rational, which requires, in turn, that they themselves be rational agents. A political community is, among other things, a way of negotiating moral differences among people. The political community is therefore not just a community of things that have moral *worth*; it is a community of entities capable of having moral *views*. If trees and mountains were said to have moral views, it would be a kind of fiction (along the lines Stone marks out for court proceedings) that could be put into practice only by giving other people the power to represent them in the community. But, to many in the community, that practice would appear to give those people, in effect, more than one vote in the polity. This problem worsens when we consider that there would be disputes about how to individuate the natural "citizens"—whether to count each tree as a member of the moral community, or each species of tree, or only a collective stand of trees or a forest. One way of gaining additional political clout would be to argue for strategies that admit greater numbers of natural "citizens."

This provides a significant moral reason not to adopt the kind of nonanthropocentric political philosophy advocated by some environmental philosophers. Some other general methodological considerations should also incline us away from a nonanthropocentric political philosophy. One is a principle of parsimony. I have argued in previous chapters that we should avoid making awkward, not easily defended metaphysical claims about how natural phenomena acquire moral value. Similarly, it makes sense to steer clear of awkward, not easily defended claims about how natural phenomena come to be the subject of public policy. A principle of parsimony guides us to assert that both of these matters happen through people: it is through people—valuers—that things acquire value, and it is through people—entities that can come together to work out value differences— that those entities come to be the subject of public policy.

Another methodological problem with trying to develop a theory that accords nature political status is that, even supposing we can figure out how to individuate the "natural" citizens, we seem to have a chance of doing that only with respect to natural states of affairs in the environment. The strategy offers no help in thinking through the political discourse concerning *human* nature or nature in the agricultural context. And, to the extent that we see these three categories of problems as structurally similar to each other, insofar as they all concern the moral status of changing natural states of affairs, it gives reason for skepticism about a political solution that accords citizenship to some natural states of affairs and not others.

A third consideration is that, however much dispute there is about the existing, anthropocentric accounts, and however difficult it is to ground policy concerning nature in these frameworks, still, we probably stand a better chance of making headway on these issues by accepting a familiar starting point than by ripping things up and trying to start over again with a new and even more controversial political philosophy.

I shall assume, at least as a starting point, that we should investigate how moral concerns about nature can be taken up into public policy and political discourse within some familiar political philosophical frameworks. In the following sections, I outline and discuss the implications for concerns about nature of Rawls's widely influential political philosophy, which holds that government should be neutral on many moral questions, and the positions of two of Rawls's critics: William Galston, who holds that a liberal society should actively promote a conception of the good but only a relatively limited, "thin" one, and Michael Sandel, who holds that policy should be based squarely on morality.

RAWLSIAN NEUTRALITY

According to one school of thought in liberal political philosophy, government should strive to maintain neutrality on a wide swath of moral questions. Rawls has been one of the leading proponents of this view. Rawls's view of neutrality starts from two key points. One is the principle of legitimacy mentioned earlier, according to which a state's political decisions are legitimate only when they can be justified to the citizens—that is, when they are made in accordance with reasons that the citizens can be expected to accept. A society that operates by this principle is more likely to be stable. It is also morally preferable, since it conforms as closely as practicable to the ideal of collective self-rule, which itself promotes the values of autonomy and respect for others.[5]

The other key starting point is the fact of philosophical disagreement. On many religious, metaphysical, and moral issues—the stuff of what Rawls calls "comprehensive doctrines"—people simply disagree. Perhaps the notion of a "comprehensive doctrine" is something of a misnomer, insofar as it suggests a more thoroughly thought-through and internally consistent, perhaps even mutually supporting, set of beliefs than many people probably have. A person's moral beliefs, metaphysical beliefs, religious beliefs, and beliefs about the way the world works probably do not form single balls of wax, and, infact, that they cannot all be easily deduced from each other is part of what makes pluralism unsurprising. Indeed, maybe it makes pluralism productive and even innately attractive for many people; pluralism is a product of the difficulty of making sense of life, a helpful resource in working though the quandaries of one's own life, a testament to the creativity of human beings, and part and parcel of a rich society.

It is also the fact of pluralism that makes the principle of legitimacy an interesting and significant constraint. If everyone were in perfect agreement, governmental decisions would always accord with the citizens' comprehensive doctrines. Given disagreement, the challenge is to promote the ideal of collective self-rule when the collected selves have different and at times incompatible ideas about what the rules should be, and to promote respect for others when others disagree with you about matters of deep mutual concern.

Rawls does not argue that governments must accord with *everyone's* beliefs, however. On core moral issues (those pertaining to autonomy and the basic moral equality of all people, for example) and on core principles of reasoning (relying on evidence and drawing conclusions logically), a liberal society is not neutral. Rawls calls these core matters the "political values"[6] or the "values of public reason."[7] A liberal society insists on them and rejects comprehensive doctrines that are inconsistent with them. It therefore accepts only a "reasonable pluralism"—that is, it accepts only doctrines that are consistent with public reason. It does not aim to offer what critics sometimes characterize as a "view from nowhere"—a view that stands above any particular set of moral commitments. It *is* a moral view.

But a "reasonable" pluralism still leaves, Rawls argues, considerable room for variation among comprehensive doctrines. Two people can affirm the values of public reason while endorsing incompatible religious positions or different views of the metaphysical status of values, for example. Moreover, they can manage to work together on the basis of what they *do* hold in common. The different parts of a comprehensive doctrine need not all be maintained together. People can sometimes bracket a disagreement by acknowledging that they elaborate and explain their core moral positions in different ways. And elaborations are not always required. If I affirm the basic moral equality of all people, I am unlikely to be asked *why* I hold that belief. (But if I assert that the Bible is the only proper basis for good public policy making, I should expect that question.)

The basic shape of the solution Rawls recommends is to rely on this idea that there are common elements—amounting to what Rawls calls an "overlapping consensus"—running through different (but reasonable) comprehensive doctrines. Rawls believes that the overlapping consensus comprises the political values. Outside the overlapping consensus, but within the pale of values tolerable within a liberal state, lie many other value questions. The political values provide some inroads into questions about the human good—it will include some degree of tolerance of alternative lifestyles, for example—but rich answers to these questions lie outside the political values. Here, too, lie answers to questions about the human relationship to nature and the moral status of nature. Government can and should, in the liberal conception, tolerate variation in these views. Further, if endorsing a view implies the suppression of others, then policy also ought avoid that endorsement.

Nonetheless, exactly how policy should relate to values outside but consistent with the political values is complex because Rawls overlays the distinction between political values and nonpolitical values with another distinction—that between the values that undergird policy making for what he calls "the basic structure of society" (which includes "such fundamental questions as who has the right to vote, or what religions are to be tolerated, or who is to be assured fair equality of opportunity, or to hold property"[8]) and the values that may be appealed to on other aspects of policy, such as funding for the arts and sciences. We should restrict ourselves to the political values when making policy relevant to the basic structure of society, but we may loosen this requirement when policy takes up other issues. Rawls suggests that the political values remain especially important for policy on these other issues but that they are not the entire story. On these "other cases," Rawls writes, "it is usually highly desirable to settle political questions by invoking the values of public reason. Yet it may not always be so."[9] The human relationship to nature is not part of the basic structure of society and is not among the fundamental questions that must be resolved by means of public reason: "the status of the natural world and our proper relation to it is not a constitutional essential or a basic question of justice."

Rawls himself is rather vague about how state policy on nonbasic but important issues relates to nonpolitical but reasonable values. The one really clear point is that government should permit the establishment of private, voluntary associations—churches, scientific associations, sports leagues, poets' societies, and so on—that have wide leeway to set their own rules and promote nonpolitical but reasonable values. They will be bound by public reason in some ways—a church should not be permitted to forcibly prevent members from leaving the church and joining some other church, for example—but not in all their activities: a church could require, as a condition of membership, that members be wealthy enough to donate money to the church.

The real difficulties arise when we consider whether *state* policy on nonbasic issues may rest on nonpolitical reasons. Rawls writes, for example, that the human relationship to nature "is a matter in regard to which citizens can vote their nonpolitical values and try to convince other citizens accordingly."[10] Thus, Rawls suggests that a degree of majoritarianism comes into play: those policies that get the most votes may carry the day (assuming that the underlying political processes are structured in a way that adheres to the political values). A more limited version of Rawls's account is developed by Thomas Murray and Peter Murray, in a paper that takes up the scope of legitimate public policy for human enhancement in sport. They accept Rawls's suggestion that government policy on nonbasic issues need not be limited by the political values, but they stop short of pure majoritarianism and elaborate on Rawls's comment that citizens may "try to convince other citizens" to accept certain nonpolitical values. They suppose, that is, that policy on nonbasic issues must still be justifiable to the citizens—just not necessarily on the basis of the political values alone. The key insight, they argue, is that citizens can deliberate together on the basis of the political values only if they have "moral powers" that would allow them to develop a broader and richer sense of the good than is specified by the political values alone,[11] and it is therefore one of the goals of government policy making to ensure the existence of a wide variety of practices and pursuits "that encourage the development and exercise" of citizens' moral powers.[12] There is "no duty to promote any one specific pursuit," but if a persuasive case can be made that a pursuit squares with, or is even conducive to, a Rawlsian conception of a just society, then the state may legitimately support that pursuit, even if the persuasive case does not rely solely on the political values. This approach will lead toward a case-by-case analysis of policy proposals.

A still more limited account is proposed by Robert Streiffer and Thomas Hedemann in a paper on the implications of Rawlsian political theory for food policy concerning genetically modified organisms. Streiffer and Hedemann distinguish between kinds of "neutrality." Policy on any topic, they acknowledge, should be neutral *in intent*: it should not be crafted specifically to forbid or discourage any reasonable comprehensive doctrine.[13] At least on matters that do not pertain to the basic structure of society, however, policy may sometimes not achieve neutrality of *effect*: a decision to install a streetlight or close a road may make it harder for some people to get to church, but still be acceptable. Whether it is will again depend on a case-by-case analysis—on how great the benefit of the policy is, how great the effect on some comprehensive doctrines is, how much the values in question matter to the people who hold them, how many people hold those values, and so on. By contrast, policies that concern the basic structure should not have the effect of making it more difficult for citizens to continue to live by a particular comprehensive doctrine. The stakes are greatest here: if these policies favored one or another comprehensive doctrine, their effect would likely be very great. Additionally, the *implications* would also be great: adopting such a policy move would imply that the affected doctrine does not have equal status in the society.

There are real discrepancies among these different accounts of the extent to which nonpolitical values may ground policy on matters outside the basic structure, and fully resolving them would require a longer trek into higher elevations of political philosophy than I can undertake here. I shall assume that the straightforward majoritarian approach Rawls appears to toy with is not right. It seems to stray too far from the principle of government neutrality on rich moral conceptions. If citizens may vote their values on nonbasic issues, then a simple majority may effectively exclude an alternative position. There are also reasons to wonder whether majoritarianism is adequately tempered by the reasons Murray and Murray give for thinking that government ought to support some "practices and pursuits" that lie outside the basic structure of society. No attempt to persuade other citizens that a given practice fits nicely within or even furthers the goals of a just society will persuade everybody that it is more deserving of support than other practices that might be supported; a majoritarian element therefore seems unavoidable in the decision to lend it support.

The critical question is whether government support for one comprehensive doctrine always implies the rejection of alternative doctrines. Does providing support for the arts necessarily imply that the state has sided with comprehensive doctrines in which the arts are valued and rejected doctrines in which the arts are frowned on as frivolous? Perhaps this depends in part, again, on the details—on what kind and level of support is provided, on what the implications are of withholding the support, on whether support for the practices and pursuits of competing doctrines is also provided. The Murrays note that there is no duty to support any one specific pursuit and that those interested in alternative pursuits are free to make their case for support and to institutionalize those pursuits alongside those for which the Murrays argue. In short, they want to stop short of permitting government endorsement. The conclusion toward which they are driving seems to be that government should offer support to positions supported by significant portions of its citizens, insofar as is necessary to carve out space within which the citizens can pursue reasonable comprehensive doctrines.

MINIMAL PERFECTIONISM

The Murrays' development of Rawls's account raises the question of whether liberalism should endorse a limited kind of "perfectionism": to what degree, that is, should a liberal state promote a particular conception of the good? A liberal state should promote the political values. Should it also encourage its citizens to develop their own richer conceptions of the good, as set out in various comprehensive doctrines? The answer to this question is clearer in the alternative account of liberalism offered by William Galston. On its face, Galston's open embrace of a kind of perfectionism should also be more amenable than Rawls's to incorporating particular moral views about the human relationship to nature into state policy.

Galston describes his position as a "minimal perfectionism": the account of the good that should inform state policy making "both defines a range of normal, decent human functioning and falls short of defining a full way of life."[14] It is a "thin" account of the good, leaving "very substantial room for individual choice and diversity,"[15] even though it is thick enough, Galston argues, to rule out some alternative accounts of the good that a nonliberal state might endorse. It is also not a exhaustively *broad* account of the good: it "does not constitute the totality of morally basic considerations either for individual action or for social policy."[16] The concepts of desert and equality, for example, are not part of it. Further, in spite of being limited both in depth and in breadth, it will remain essentially contested, in W. B. Gallie's sense, because it can be specified in varying ways and no one way of specifying it can be proven true in light of still deeper moral insights.

Galston suggests, then (although noting that no account of the good can be "hard and fast"), that a liberal account of the good will incorporate a number of "key dimensions."[17] It will hold that:

- life is good, although it is not always an overriding good;
- human beings are typically born with certain physical, cognitive, and social capacities, lack or loss of which is generally a misfortune and development of which is good;
- human beings tend to form interests and purposes, and it is generally good both to be able to form them and then to seek to fulfill them;
- freedom is "an indispensable element of each individual's good";[18]
- although a liberal society will not endorse a life of the mind over a life of say, faith, rationality is good;
- society—"the network of significant relations we establish with others"—is an important element of the good; and
- finally, pure subjective satisfaction—pleasure, security—counts for something.

The list does not include any general claims about the human relationship to nature. Possibly, the list is relevant to claims specifically about the human relationship to *human* nature, since it stipulates that certain naturally attributes of human beings are part of the human good. As to the nature of nonhuman species or the environment at large, the most that could be said is that an individual might place that relationship among the "interests and purposes" fulfillment of which would be a key dimension of the good. A public theory of the good, however, does not specifically embrace that possibility.

Perhaps this is only to be expected, since we are considering so far only an account of the human good, and the human relationship to nature seems to fall into the category of "other moral considerations" that can figure both in individual action and public policy. An account of the human good is the starting point, however. That account, augmented by a principle that each person's good should be of equal weight in forming public policy, provides the basis for a theory of public purposes and a theory of public claims: the overall purpose of a liberal state is collaboratively "to create and sustain circumstances within which individuals may pursue—and to the greatest possible extent achieve—their good," and insofar as this purpose is pursued collaboratively, individuals make claims on each other. Galston identifies three kinds of claims: "those arising from the bare fact of membership in the community (need); those arising from contribution to the community (desert); and those arising from the voluntary individual disposition of resources in areas left undetermined by the legitimate claims of others (choice)."[19] He illustrates these categories by means of social and economic examples, but remarks that "structurally similar convictions apply in the political sphere as well."[20] The principle of equality generates a commitment to equal voting rights, for example. Need and desert generate commitments to give all people opportunities to practice citizenship but to reserve the highest political offices for those with the greatest merit. The principle of choice translates into a belief "that when fair procedures govern a sphere in which public authority may legitimately act, the outcome is to be respected."[21]

So, what is the public authority's range of legitimate action? The political version of the principle of choice seems to make room for policy on topics that might be affected by citizens' moral views about the human relationship to nature. That policy could address, for example, the disposition of the society's natural resources, food production, and medical technology—plausibly all spheres in which the public authority may legitimately take action. But still there is a question whether moral views about the human relationship to nature are legitimate *grounds* for policy in these spheres.

There are several reasons in Galston's account to maintain some skepticism about state enforcement of moral views about nature. First, the overall theory of public policy making is that it remains centered around an understanding of the human good and how best to achieve it, and human beings' moral commitments to the natural world figure in indirectly, insofar as being able to act on one's interests is part of the human good. No one standard for the relationship to nature is a necessary human interest.

A preservationist stance is but one possible view, for instance. Indeed, the considerable disagreement over what stance to take toward nature argues for keeping it out of the thin theory. Galston explains his requirement that a thin theory of the good must achieve only minimal unity and leave much room for diversity by noting that a liberal theory of the good "arises in large measure from a deep common experience of the bad."[22] "We can agree that death, wanton cruelty, slavery, poverty, malnutrition, vulnerability, and humiliation are bad without having a fully articulated unitary account of the good." A feeling of being out of step with nature does not make this list.

Nor is a particular relationship to nature flatly necessary for the human good. Preventing environmental damage that will make the world inhospitable, even uninhabitable, is necessary for any human good, but this is a practical point; Galston's list of background conditions sets *logical* parameters for a theory of the good—they are stipulations concerning the limits, bases, and general shape of a theory of the good. Also, at least in principle, severe environmental damage could be avoided in a way that squared better with an interventionist than a preservationist stance; one strategy occasionally proposed for preventing global warming, for example, is diverting sunlight by sprinkling the atmosphere with reflective materials.

Furthermore, there is some reason to think that views about the moral status of nature do not belong comfortably to "a sphere in which public authority may legitimately act." Galston cites with approval Locke's arguments for preventing the state from attempting to impose a religion on citizens (although noting that Rawlsian liberals often wrongly suppose that the arguments support keeping the state entirely out of legislating about virtue). To some degree, Locke's arguments hang on the very special, other-worldly character of religious belief. The state, being very much of this world, is not competent to assess the truth of religious belief, and the state's power of coercion is not capable of bringing about the "inward persuasion of the mind" in which "true and saving religion" consists.[23]

On the other hand, some of Locke's arguments also seem to give reason to restrict public policy concerning attitudes toward nature. An argument from what Galston calls "epistemological neutrality" is that, often, "no rational adjudication is possible among competing claims."[24] This consideration would surely apply to competing claims about the preferable human relationship to nature. An argument from "rights-based neutrality" is that, as Locke puts it, "Human beings enter into civil society to attain and protect nonmoral goods: goods of the body and external possessions . . . , [and] the sovereign's legitimate sway extends no farther than this initial grant."[25] To the extent that nature is considered a human good that humans want to attain and protect, then the state may impose constraints on its use, but the view that nature is *intrinsically* good, however, may not provide a legitimate basis for policy, so that policy based only or primarily on that view would not be legitimate. Finally, the state may adopt a position of neutrality for prudential reasons, insofar as attempts to enforce a uniform view tend to be counterproductive, leading only toward deeper division.

Galston believes that liberalism requires not only an account of the public good but also of public virtue: a liberal society can function only when citizens exhibit "individual self-discipline and self-restraint." Yet the writ here is to foster a collective endeavor to create and maintain circumstances in which individuals can pursue the good as they somewhat variously understand it, and the scope of legitimate state action on moral matters is therefore limited. Liberalism should promote moral principles and virtues that foster this endeavor, and it should be "wary" of attempts to translate "personal moral sentiment" into coercive public policy. "[S]entiments of the form 'X is unnatural, disgusting, ungodly (or whatever)'" do not alone provide a basis for legal proscription of anything judged unacceptable by those standards.[26]

In short, Galston's minimal perfectionism seeks to go further than Rawls's liberal neutrality in permitting government enaction of rich moral views, but it, too, stops short of declaring unambiguously that moral judgments about the human relationship to nature may lead directly to legal enforcement. If the overarching goal of the liberal state is "to create and sustain circumstances within which individuals may pursue—and to the greatest possible extent achieve—their good," then moral views about the human relationship to nature lie in a contested domain, in that they are arguably but not obviously part of the citizens' good and stand in tension with other citizens' views in a way that may lead the state to treat them gingerly. If "creating and sustaining circumstances" that allow citizens to live by these values requires active government support, then the government should probably provide that support to the extent it can without overriding other citizens' views. As with Rawlsian liberalism, we are left with a picture in which government ought to act positively but circumspectly to carve out space for alternative views.

COMMUNITARIANISM

Michael Sandel's "republican" approach—often described as a "communitarian" approach, although Sandel himself expresses discomfort with the term—offers a contrasting slant to the issue of how views about the human relationship to nature might be taken up into policy. Sandel rests his position on a rejection of Rawslian liberal neutrality on moral questions. For Sandel, there is no general distinction between morality and public policy: he quotes approvingly Aristotle's maxim that "any polis which is truly so called, and is not merely one in name, must devote itself to the end of encouraging goodness. Otherwise," he goes on to explain, "a political association sinks into a mere alliance.... Otherwise, too, law becomes a mere covenant—or (in the phrase of the Sophist Lycophron) 'a guarantor of men's rights against one another'—instead of being, as it should be, a rule of life such as will make the members of a polis good and just."[27]

Within American political life, Sandel argues, the liberal view of individual liberty—which he characterizes as amounting to freedom from coercion and requiring government neutrality on moral questions—is of fairly recent origin. The country was actually founded on a "republican" view of liberty, in which liberty consisted partly in participation in the civic life of a self-governing community. Participating in the community's self-governance requires that one possess what Sandel calls the "civic virtues"—a sense of belonging to the civic life, "a concern for the whole, a moral bond with the community whose fate is at stake."[28] The civic virtues also include a capacity to deliberate about the common good and a willingness to put the common good above one's own interests.[29] Acquiring them requires that citizens undergo a kind of character education—people must be trained to participate in the society—and the ultimate responsibility for this training falls to society itself: "The republican conception of freedom ... requires a formative politics, a politics that cultivates in citizens the qualities of character self-government requires."[30] Thus, government cannot be neutral toward the moral positions its citizens settle upon.

Government policy making therefore is fundamentally a matter of making moral assessments. The question of whether research on human embryos should receive federal funding turns straightforwardly on the social benefits of the research and the moral status of human embryos, and their status is not a matter to be left to religion or to private citizens, but is to be worked out publicly.[31] The reason homosexual unions ought to be permitted is not that homosexuality is a private matter—a domain where the state may not tread—but that homosexual unions promote many of the same values that conventional marriages promote.[32] The issue of whether citizens should be allowed to seek assisted suicide depends on how to balance "the claims of compassion," which in cases of excruciating and terminal illness may call on us to "hasten death," against the reverence for life—assisted suicide is not a private decision, and citizens do not have a right to it.[33]

Sandel stops short of saying that government should make *all* of an individual's moral decisions, however. Some decisions can be made only by individuals. Sandel argues, for example, that government should protect the free exercise of religion on grounds that "religious belief, as character-istically practiced in a particular society, produces ways of being and acting that are worthy of honor and appreciation—either because they are admi-rable in themselves or because they foster qualities of character that make good citizens."[34] Sandel is somewhat obscure about the extent of religious liberty. He does not say whether any particular religion might be promoted over others, if it turned out that adherents to the religion had better quali-ties of character than others. He also does not say whether the free exercise of nonreligion would be protected. The concept of religious liberty, as most people understand it, seems to include liberty to practice atheism, but if religious belief produces better character, then atheism would apparently produce worse character. A charitable reading, however, would be that a fairly broad religious liberty is protected.

So, how to think about the human relationship to nature? On the one hand, Sandel has explicitly taken up the question biotechnology poses con-cerning the human relationship to nature, and he apparently holds that a careful moral analysis points toward good policy. For example, the prob-lem with allowing parents to genetically enhance their children is that it conflicts with some of the goods that are part of parenting—the norms of unconditional love of one's children and of openness to the develop-ment of unexpected traits and qualities in them.[35] In general, medical bio-technology, with its promise of curing disease and extending the human lifespan, promotes a hubris and idolatrousness that can be at odds with religious norms, and that conflict (Sandel apparently holds) may inform our understanding of the best ethical and legal stance toward biotechnol-ogies. Technologies to enhance human beings could also undermine the virtue of social solidarity among people because they would lead to distinc-tions between the enhanced and the unenhanced that would tend to drive citizens apart from each other.

On the other hand, there might be reasons to think that government should not rush to endorse positions concerning the human relationship to nature. One consideration is that the ideal of preserving nature does not seem to fall squarely within the range of values that, in Sandel's frame-work, should be promoted by the state. The values that clearly warrant pro-motion are those that Sandel groups under the heading of civic virtues, which are capacities and stances that contribute to a well-functioning com-munity. This will not be a narrowly bounded part of the moral life; one way or another, a focus on the civic virtues will give the state warrant to promote a wide range of moral positions: a well-functioning community requires deliberation about and pursuit of the common good, and most moral issues will bear in some way on the common good. Some, however, will be more vital to the well-functioning community than others. Sandel identifies a willingness to put the common good above one's own as vital, and a capacity to deliberate well about the common good would undoubtedly be essential. Society should presumably work hard to promote these virtues. Many other virtues, such as the virtues of managing one's time and developing one's talents, vital though they might be to individuals, are not quite as vital to society and would not warrant the same level of robust promotion as the civic virtues. Moving still further from moral categories that are vital to society would be more idiosyncratic standards. A Thoreau-like willingness to make one's own way—to think new thoughts and buck the tide—counts, for some, as a type to be admired and emulated (it might be a moral ideal, as described in Chapter 3). Society should probably tolerate this standard. A citizen could live by it while manifesting civic virtues. And society might be enriched by people who live their lives this way, insofar as it appeals to some citizens, contributes to cultural diversity, and fosters creativity and leadership. But it is not at all clear that society should *encourage* citizens to live this way. A society of such people might almost be dysfunctional. And there is an almost diametrically contrasting standard. Many will cleave instead to a deep social connectedness and belonging and conformity to existing social patterns—compliance over originality, pulling together over bucking the tide. This standard, too, has clear social benefits.

Moral views about the human relationship to nature seem to be the kind of moral position that is not vital for the good of the community. They have to do with individual commitments more than with social benefit. They are not integral to the development of a well-functioning society; indeed, a conservative or preservationist stance toward nature can foster behavior that stands over against the likely good of the community—reluctance about developing new technologies and a nod to environment preservation and species protection over economic progress. (Of course, one kind of environmentalism—one oriented toward protection of the public health and of resources that have public benefits—would provide a civic benefit and might fall within the ambit of civic virtue.) The contrasting standards—that of the engineer pushing a technology along and building new devices or the developer making the best use of natural resources—are also acceptable, insofar as civic welfare is the goal. Furthermore, to encourage the central civic virtue of deliberating well about the good, the state ought to make a point of leaving *room* for deliberation, and unless the good is already quite well understood, that deliberation ought to be not only about how to achieve the good, but also about what the good is—what values go into it. Thus, the state should hesitate to try to specify moral values that are not vital to its own flourishing.

In the communitarian picture, too, then, it seems that government policy would seek to make room for both nature-preserving and nature-improving moral stances, supporting each insofar as it can without eliminating the other. It would evince a kind of neutrality, in other words: it would seek to protect them by allowing citizens to live by them.

STATE POLICY AND PERSONAL IDEALS

The attractiveness of some degree of state neutrality with respect to moral views about the human relationship to nature is heightened, for all of the positions overviewed here, if the proposal floated in the previous chapter is on the mark and those moral views should be understood as *ideals*—as standards that individuals seek to live by but that as a *moral* matter (not merely as a political matter) are not seen as socially enforceable. Individuals who particularly cherish one ideal undoubtedly want to promote it, but whether and how state resources should be spent promoting it is very far from clear, and its *promotion* should come up somewhere shy of *enforcement*. We do not expect complete agreement on ideals, and, in fact, the multiplicity of ideals contributes to the richness of society—it is itself part of the social good.

A second general sort of consideration that might be offered for governmental neutrality is that the ideal of nature is, in at least one sense, a quasi-religious orientation. It is similar to religious belief in that it gives meaning and value to a person's life. Honoring the ideal is a way of giving one's life worthwhile content. But this is an internal orientation of the individual: it requires that the individual be deliberating about and committing him- or herself to the ideal. It depends therefore on endorsement rather than enforcement. It cannot simply be imposed on a person; it must be taken up internally. (The ideal of nature might also be religious in a stronger sense, in that it might be interwoven with claims about the ultimate reality of the cosmos or the existence of God. Perhaps the ideal of nature was inextricably bound up with metaphysical beliefs for John Muir, for example, who saw in nature evidence of God's goodness. But I am leaving this sense aside here.)

Finally, the comparison to religious beliefs suggests a pragmatic reason to be wary of governmental promotion of the ideal of nature, which is simply that the community might benefit from tolerating a diversity of views on a subject that does, after all, lend itself to a diversity of views and over-laps in some measure with religious belief. Sandel makes this kind of point about governmental toleration of diverse religious beliefs: "upholding religious liberty could still be justified as a way of avoiding the civil strife that can result when church and state are too closely intertwined."[36]

THE PUBLIC GOOD AND RESPECT
FOR PRIVATE DIFFERENCES

This survey, quick and limited though it is, suggests the attractiveness of a *more or less* liberal account of government neutrality, at least for the issue of citizens' values concerning the human relationship to nature. Government should carve out a space for those values but should come up well shy of enforcing them. The question, then, is how to carve out a space in which those who cherish a natural states of affairs—who heed the "call of the wild"—can live by their values. How should the state make it possible for people to live by their values but avoid actually enforcing values? What does this mean for public policy? In the remainder of this chapter, I try to make good on my promise at the beginning to show that public policy should go somewhat further than the liberal principle of neutrality might, on its face, seem to allow—at the very least, further than some critics of it have thought it allows. I want to argue that the liberal policy of neutrality is not the same as a hands-off, leave-everyone-alone policy. I want to play off the image of *carving out* a space and argue that the liberal state should take a more supportive stance toward those values than it would if it merely *left matters alone*; that the goal of the state should not be to vacate the area outside Rawls's political values but to create it, through positive but cautious intervention.

To fix our options, it may help to identify the extreme ends of the spectrum of possibilities for government support for moral values—meaning not just what Rawls calls the core liberal values or what Galston calls a thin conception of the good, but an array of values that would make up a broader or richer understanding of the good, a set of values among which a particular stance on the human relationship to nature might find its place. At one end is the possibility of enforcing allegiance. If preservation is deemed the morally better stance toward the human relationship to nature, then government could require any behavior that it deems accords with that behavior and outlaw behavior that is deemed to conflict with it. The government's power to enforce values would be akin to government's power in a theocracy to require adherence to a particular religion. Perhaps

declarations of allegiance to nature preservation could be made mandatory. This could make for some wonderful nature preserves—imagine
imposing strict nature-preservationist behavior on the citizens of South
Dakota to create a Tallgrass Prairie National Park throughout the state,
with all off-road vehicles prohibited and herds of millions of bison allowed
to migrate through the yards of any citizens who remain in the state. But
this option would surely violate the principle of neutrality.

At the other end is the hands-off, leave-everyone-alone stance, according to which the state should allow people who have preservationist values
to act on their values but no more: such values can be supported only in
the private sphere, by citizens acting on their own behalf. Citizens would
be let alone, free to choose and live by their values as best they can, and
to muster support for their values through mechanisms available to citizens in an open society—by advocating for their views, by coming together
in organizations like The Nature Conservancy to purchase land and create
nature preserves, and by, in effect, marketing their positions via movies,
television shows, and the like. The extent of government activity should be
to step away from projects that imply support for some values over others.
Government support for moral values outside the core liberal values should
be modeled on how government support for religion is often understood in
the United States, as a sharp breach.

What I hope to show, then, is that some sort of middle position between
these extremes satisfies the requirements of neutrality well enough. I am
agnostic as to whether, in making this claim, I am sliding away from Rawls
toward Galston, or simply explicating Rawls's own true position and correcting a common misinterpretation.

One straightforward point to put on the table is that middling positions between the extremes are known to be possible, given that current practice is, in fact, somewhere in the middle. Government provides
support for a variety of richer conceptions of the good through various
funding mechanisms, for example. There is more than a little publicly supported science, for example, that is basically science for the sake of science—science that seems worth undertaking not because it brings such
great benefits but because of the intrinsic value widely found in learning
and knowledge. Space exploration, the Hubble telescope, paleontology,
archeology, and some kinds of biological research (say, of life at deep sea
vents) all receive federal support yet arguably are valued more because of
their contributions to knowledge than because of their contributions to
human welfare. Government also supports scholarship in the humanities
through, for example, the funding distributed by the National Endowment
for the Humanities and the work of the Woodrow Wilson International

Center for Scholars. Perhaps the classic example of government support for intrinsic values is government support for the arts, exemplified by the National Endowment for the Arts, whose overall funding reflects support for a rather generic valuation of arts and arts education and whose funding for particular projects can support particular values that are reflected in artists' work. Government support for the arts also includes state-level grants and local funding devoted to theaters, museums, concerts, and so on. Federal funding also tacitly supports all sorts of values through the tax deduction offered to philanthropic gifts. If someone backs up the value they find in philosophical examination of issues in bioethics by making a gift to The Hastings Center (as I highly recommend), that value receives a modicum of government support.

Government funding is a modestly coercive way of supporting a value. It does not mandate anyone's endorsement of it, and it does not restrict anyone's range of activity, but it compels them, in effect, to give money to it. Currently, policy goes beyond this degree of coercion to incorporate government *restrictions* on private citizens' activities and differential extension of special rights and privileges. Zoning laws may be used to shape the communities we live in, reflecting values both about human relationships and, sometimes, the human relationship to nature. And, finally, arriving squarely at the topic taken up in this chapter, the Endangered Species Act, the Wilderness Act, the Wild and Scenic Rivers Act, the National Wildlife Refuge System, and probably the National Park System reflect support for the intrinsic value many find in the natural world, and many state and local efforts, of course, follow suit.

Of course, the fact that government policy does not now conform to the hands-off stance does not show that the hands-off stance is not required by neutrality, unless we also stipulate that current policy conforms to neutrality. The most that can be said is this: to the degree that the liberal theory of neutrality is meant to be descriptive of the kind of stance that typifies contemporary government policy in the United States toward rich moral conceptions, it should avoid committing itself to the hands-off stance, and, to the degree that we are pleased that government policy takes up those conceptions (with quibbles possible, of course), we should avoid endorsing a hands-off stance.

A second point against the hands-off stance is that it is actually impracticable because it relies on an untenable distinction between *promoting welfare* and *supporting a particular group's values*. The hands-off stance supposes that promotion of the general welfare must be the primary rationale for supporting science, arts, and the humanities, funding zoos and museums, building parks and stadiums to create opportunities for recreation, and protecting the environment. Possibly, some of these investments also play a small role in inculcating the civic virtues that Rawls, Galston, and Sandel all discuss, but in some cases that will be a stretch. It is a stretch, in particular, for measures to protect the natural environment. Any government support for environmental causes would have to be grounded on claims about human welfare: the Endangered Species Act is defensible, one might say, because biodiversity can foster the development of useful drugs and industrial materials, and the Wilderness Act and the National Park System because they provide pleasure and promote physical activity.

But human welfare cannot be singled out as the sole basis for government support in these examples. In the first place, that strategy is often simply disingenuous. Preserving biodiversity *in general* may help lead to new drugs and materials, but, in many specific cases, we know enough to relax the rule, if the rule has only that justification. Preserving spotted owls is unlikely to produce new medical insights, for example. And although wildernesses certainly provide a form of recreation, the very concept of a wilderness ensures that not too many people can partake of that recreation at any one time; turning the land over to snowmobile or all-terrain-vehicle races would be more productive, if the justification is promotion of human delight. Second, in very many cases, human welfare cannot really be disentangled from intrinsic values. Typically, what makes something pleasurable or entertaining depends on other, richer values. A play in a football game or a sequence in a ballet performance is electrifying only if one buys into some of the values that football or ballet is designed to celebrate. One must appreciate grit, strength, and all-out determination to get any thrill out of the controlled violence that is football. One must find some value in nature in order to think that canoeing in a wilderness is an enjoyable kind of recreation.

In short, to speak of justifying public projects *solely* because of how they promote human welfare is to endorse an implausibly narrow, utilitarian understanding of welfare. Human welfare is informed by other values, such that it is impossible to aim only at welfare without also supporting, in some way, some of the values dear to particular groups of people. In some way, one endorses some richer values dear to particular subsets of the larger population. Policy aimed at promoting "welfare" therefore frequently also threatens to promote values that seem to fall outside the core liberal values. One can try, for example, to explain governmental decisions to set places aside by talking blandly about "outdoor recreation," but, in fact, outdoor recreation will tend to reflect one or another view of how humans should be related to the outdoors. If liberal government is to make good on its "reasonable," consensus goal of advancing human welfare, then it must somehow engage with particular intrinsic values.

To be sure, there are some topics for which a much thinner conception of the good is more tenable. Every citizen can plausibly be said to benefit, regardless of their conception of the good, from public health interventions that reduce threats from disease and national defense measures that significantly lessen the possibility of foreign invasion, for example. For somewhat similar reasons, health policy, education, consumer protections, and trade and economic policy are at least candidates for a purely utilitarian conception of the good. Some level of decent health can be presented as a good necessary to achieve other goods, for example, and the overall economic strength and stability of a country can be described as benefitting everybody in it.

Of course, government policy is mostly not thought to be limited to these domains; it also enacts policy that promotes recreation, home ownership, marriage, and charitable giving, for example. Even within these domains, however, a thin characterization of benefit may be more elusive than initially appears. The very idea that health policy, public education, and consumer protections would be matters on which government should enact policy, on behalf of citizens, implies a fairly strong commitment to collective action and orientation toward community, and that commitment (at the strength necessary to support these policies) is not itself part of every "reasonable" account of the good. Also, government policy that promotes trade and growth will ineluctably blend into policy that favors a life dedicated to participating actively in trade and economic activity—again, not part and parcel of every conception of the good. Moreover, as government proceeds to enact policy on such matters, the question is not so much whether health per se is part of every conception of the good, but whether this or that kind of health-promoting intervention is part of the good, and disagreement naturally grows as the decisions become more fine-grained. Also, of course, these questions will arise not simply as questions about whether some policy is desirable, but about whether it is more or less desirable than other possible policies that compete with it for government resources. What we are left with, then, is that for some domains of government policy, we can get somewhat further with a utilitarian rationale than we can when addressing other domains, but for none or almost none is the understanding of welfare completely disentangled from richer conceptions of the good, and on many other matters that are already widely considered acceptable topics for government policy, a thin conception of the good looks quite inadequate. If liberal government is to make good on its "reasonable," consensus goal of advancing human welfare, then it must provide some support for particular intrinsic values.

A third consideration telling against the strict, hands-off reading of neutrality is that, given a capitalist economy, a strict hands-off stance would sometimes amount to choosing sides, since it would have the inevitable consequence that some values lose out. A strict hands-off stance endorses a kind of moral free market: values must duke it out among themselves, and those that are most persuasive will win over adherents, survive, and be carried forth into the world by their proponents. Government has nothing to say about which one wins. There's more than a little to be said in favor of this idea; after all, we endorse something like an intellectual free market in science—we think that ideas are supposed to beat out other ideas and attract proponents because they are better, not because their proponents are more powerful. But values do not win or lose in the same way that ideas in science do. Good ideas in science win partly because they help us get around in the world. They *make* their adherents more powerful. Values are also linked to getting around in the world, but frequently in the opposite way: they are constraints on action rather than facilitators of it. When one chooses to abide by one's values, one may even be deciding *against* one's worldly benefit.

In short, scientific advance is conducive to success in the world in a way that moral virtue is not. The moral free market contains too many exogenous factors to function properly. In particular, a moral free market is overlaid in particularly distracting ways by the economic market. Very possibly, the Protestant work ethic attracted adherents because it was conducive to worldly success, but whether it was *morally* better than alternative positions is a separate question. Surely, every parent in the United States today feels, at times, a clash between work ethic—productivity, accountability, seeing a job through to the end even if it means putting in extra hours— and commitment to family. Bioethics, as a field for scholarly and policy work, has its roots in the clash between the value of developing products that will help treat illness—which benefits the community at large but also often aligns nicely with personal gain for the researcher—and the value of protecting the research subject's right to make informed decisions about his or her own medical care.

The question, then, is whether government may do anything to preserve or protect value positions that, lacking its support, look likely to be trampled. The argument here is that neutrality requires more support than a hands-off stance allows because if government has also established a capitalist economy, then a hands-off stance is sometimes not neutral. The exogenous factors providing incentives against moral values are easy to understand when the values at stake concern the human relationship to nature and the moral question is, "May we remake the world to suit our own ends?" There is a clash of values here, between the values of development— human welfare, individual productivity, resourcefulness—and those of a preservationist mindset, and it is clear enough which side the market is on. In such a case, neutrality is not achieved by remaining resolutely hands-off. Instead, government must do something to shore up the disadvantaged side.

There is a bit of a Catch-22 in this point, unfortunately. Some values need government support because, without it, they will tend to lose out and their adherents will be pressed to the side; but for just the same reason that they need government support they may tend to lose the political battles necessary in a democracy to gain government support. The hope must be that when people are making decisions at the level of social policy—when citizens are voting and when those elected are setting policy—they are better able to set aside the economic distractions and choose on the basis of their values. This may be a wan hope, of course. But that is the basic idea of democracy—that the free-for-all, the all-against-all, can be replaced with something more deliberative and protective of values.

A fourth and purely moral reason not to endorse the hands-off, stringently neutral version of the liberal principle of neutrality is that a deeper, more supportive engagement is necessary to adequately respect other fellow citizens. The argument here parallels a point made in the previous chapter and can be laid out swiftly: respect for others is one of the underlying principles of liberalism; indeed, the moral justification for the liberal principle of neutrality is that it is necessary in order to show proper respect for others. We show respect for others, in part, by allowing others to make, and live by, their own value positions (consistent with the liberal society), even when we do not share those values. But, sometimes, respect for a value position can require more than simply letting people fend for themselves. Sometimes we must lend them a hand.

Suppose I live in a community that deeply honors its history. I am a newcomer to the community and do not particularly share this interest in history. In fact, I think a forward-looking attitude is more to be fostered; although we can learn from the past, we should not hold it up as having any special value. While digging in the garden, though, I discover some artifacts that I believe would be extremely valuable to those in the community who share the history-valuing standpoint. I might be within my rights to dispose of the artifacts. A respectful stance toward those in my community who *would* value them, however, should incline me to save them and pass them along to the history lovers. Similarly, if I join the village board, I might vote to approve funding for a village history room in the library in order to honor the assiduous efforts of a group of village historians who have been collecting stories and artifacts that detail the community's past. If I know that some of the older residents of the community are proud of their predecessors' stories but have begun to feel that those stories are ignored and underappreciated as newer residents like me have settled in the village and changed its culture, then I am likely to see that as further reason to try to find the funding. On a national scale, the Smithsonian has roughly the same goals; some such considerations were in play in the run-up to approving the building of a National Museum of African American History and Culture. One of the goals of a government should be to honor its citizens' cultures; to honor those cultures is, in some measure, to support their values.

THE WAY FORWARD

Where do these four considerations lead? Of course, the liberal principle of neutrality has generated a broader literature than has been addressed here. The *suggestion*, however—the challenge that the argument so far presents—is that if we are to retain the principle of neutrality, then maybe we will have to opt for a rather complicated view of it. Maybe the liberal principle of neutrality means something rougher, something like this: that a liberal government should handle values that lie outside the overlapping consensus warily, but if it is to promote citizens' welfare, then it will nonetheless have to take positive measures to support those values. It should try to avoid taking sides between the richer, more controversial values held by its citizens, but it should seek to create space, create the possibilities, that allow citizens to act on those values.

This does not provide a *clean* understanding of "neutrality"; we might be left admitting that neutrality will always be in danger of slipping into policy that takes sides, and whether government policy is appropriately neutral will always be debatable. But this is simply to say that neutrality is like many other concepts that are deployed in moral thinking. It is, like the concept of nature itself, an essentially contested concept. That outcome should not lead us to conclude that the concept is useless and should be jettisoned. It also should not lead us to give up on attempts to clean it up—to draw distinctions between different kinds of values, or different kinds of justifications for them, and show that some may receive governmental support and some may not. Even if those efforts—which I have not explored here—do not resolve everything, they can still be illuminating. We will never know just what policy to adopt concerning the human relationship to nature, not simply because of abiding moral disagreements, but also because of deep-seated difficulties in the very idea of carrying out any one view by means of policy.

A quick reprise of the argument so far: Chapter 1 argued that we can sensibly talk about natural states of affairs—the concept of nature is not always so muddled as to be useless. Chapter 2 argued that valuing natural states of affairs can be a legitimate moral position. Chapter 3 suggested that the value of nature figures in our moral deliberations in a complex way, often more as a personal ideal than as a social obligation. This chapter has tried to argue that moral views about nature may legitimately be taken up in public policy, but not in such a way as to exclude competing views. Rather, public policy should aim, where it can, to carve out room in which citizens can live by their values.

So, what would it mean to "carve out a space" for the view that leaving natural states of affairs alone can be morally valuable? What would these solutions look like? Does a general stance that leaving nature alone is desirable translate into the same kind of policy solution on every issue about which it can be held? And can it be done, even in principle? Would it amount to a kind of defeat? Would those views be consigned to the periphery and be ultimately overwhelmed as the cultural mainstream churns along in whatever direction it is impelled, driven by the desire for resources and competition *of* resources that characterize social relations in a liberal society? These questions require that we treat the abstractions of this and foregoing chapters in the context of the particular social debates in which they arise.

NOTES

1. US Senator Jim Bunning, "Statement by U.S. Senator Jim Bunning, House Government Reform Hearing on Steroids and Major League Baseball," House of Representatives Committee on Oversight and Government Reform, March 17, 2005.
2. Robyn Eckersley, *Environmentalism and Political Theory: Toward an Ecocentric Approach* (Albany, N.Y.: State University of New York Press, 1992).
3. Christopher Stone, *Should Trees Have Moral Standing? Toward Legal Rights for Natural Objects* (Los Altos, Cal.: William Kaufmann, Inc., 1974).
4. John Rawls, *Political Liberalism* (New York: Columbia University Press, 1993), 217.
5. Harry Brighouse, *School Choice and Social Justice* (Oxford, U.K.: Oxford University Press, 2000), 7, 12.
6. Rawls, *Political Liberalism*, 214
7. Ibid., 215.
8. Ibid., 214.
9. Ibid., 215.
10. Ibid., 246.
11. Thomas H. Murray and Peter Murray, "Rawls, Sports, and Liberal Legitimacy," in *The Ideal of Nature: Debates about Biotechnology and the Environment*, ed. Gregory

E. Kaebnick (Baltimore, Md.: Johns Hopkins University Press, 2011), 179–99, at 186.

12. Murray and Murray, "Rawls, Sports, and Liberal Legitimacy," 189.

13. Rob Streiffer and Thomas Hedemann, "The Political Import of Intrinsic Objections to Genetically Engineered Food," *Journal of Agriculture and Environmental Ethics* 18 (2004), 191–210.

14. William A. Galston, *Liberal Purposes: Goods, Virtues, and Diversity in the Liberal State* (Cambridge, U.K.: Cambridge University Press, 1991), 177.

15. Ibid., 167.

16. Ibid., 166.

17. Ibid., 173–77.

18. Ibid., 175.

19. Ibid., 183–84.

20. Ibid., 189.

21. Ibid., 189–90.

22. Ibid., 168.

23. Ibid., 260.

24. Ibid., 259.

25. Ibid., 260.

26. Ibid., 280.

27. Michael Sandel, *Democracy's Discontent: America in Search of a Public Philosophy* (Cambridge, Mass.: Belknap Press, 1998), 7.

28. Ibid., 5.

29. Ibid., 26.

30. Ibid., 6.

31. Michael Sandel, *Public Philosophy: Essays on Morality in Politics* (Cambridge, Mass.: Harvard University Press, 2006), 117ff.

32. Sandel, *Public Philosophy*, 137.

33. Ibid., 116.

34. Ibid., 257.

35. Michael Sandel, *The Case Against Perfectionism: Ethics in the Age of Genetic Engineering* (Cambridge, Mass.: Belknap Press, 2009), 85ff.

36. Sandel, *Public Philosophy*, 257.

CHAPTER 5

Nature Naturalized

Wilderness and Wildlife

I grew up in east Tennessee, in a valley between the Cumberland Mountains and the Smoky Mountains. The Smokies were, in my parochial view, the crown jewel of the Appalachian chain, blessed with the highest peaks in the eastern United States, the biggest trees, the greatest biodiversity, and a decent chunk of the last remaining old-growth eastern forest. They also had the most salamanders. For me, growing up, the Smokies were the place to go to be connected with nature. I went as often as I could. I was fascinated by everything I learned about them. It was almost a place of worship for me. It was a place of wilderness, of nature escaping the march of malls and highways.

But, of course, I knew that the Smokies are not pure wilderness. They have been altered by humans in all sorts of ways. Many species have been eliminated by humans, from panthers and the Carolina parakeet to the American chestnut (although old stumps still send up shoots); some have been introduced (such as the European wild boar, which eats many native plants, and Asian kudzu, "the vine that ate the South"); and a few that were lost have been reintroduced (the red wolf, unsuccessfully, and elk, successfully). Almost all of the land now "preserved" in the national park was logged, and much of it has been used as pasture. There were a number of small communities throughout it, roads and railroads crisscrossed it, and, of course, there are roads, trails, campgrounds, and various facilities throughout the park today.

Is it "wilderness" at all? Is it even really "natural"? This is a broad problem, of course. A similar question has arisen about the Amazon rain forest, widely thought of as one of the world's last remaining true wildernesses, a place that is simply inhospitable for human civilization according to the dominant view among the last generation of anthropologists. People were known to have lived there, but only in small hunter-gatherer communities. Agriculture on a large scale was thought impossible, and, without the agricultural revolution, there could be no division of labor between farmers and tradesmen and therefore no complex civilization. An up and coming generation of scholars apparently argues otherwise, however; these anthropologists claim to have discovered evidence of huge fields and waterworks, evidence apparently that a vastly larger population once existed in the region. There may have been cities. Forests were felled; rivers diverted. The soil was improved in huge swaths of land by adding charcoal. A place that appears to be pristine nature—almost entirely free of human influence—is perhaps not, after all.

The first chapter argued that the concept of "nature" need not be defined so sharply that we can always tell what states of affairs count as natural and what do not, and the account we give of its meaning need not be thought of as arising independently of human convention (in both these ways, it is like many other morally significant concepts). We can, rather, allow that the line between natural and nonnatural is indistinct, and we can allow that where the line is drawn is partly dependent on convention. But I have not yet shown how these claims work out in practice—how "nature," understood to function along the lines I have delineated, can still be useful. If the concept is too fuzzy, or changes shape with shifting convention too readily, we might yet end up rejecting it.

This chapter takes up the challenge: it tries to show that "nature" can, in fact, be workable, and, in keeping with the thrust of the argument so far, it will do so by considering the role of the concept in debates about environmental protection, which provide a useful starting point for a larger examination of the concept of nature. Insofar as "nature" involves a distinction of some sort between what is human and what arises independently of humanity, the concept must work in debates about the environment—the world *around* humans—if it is to work anywhere, and showing how it works in these debates might provide some insight that might be useful for thinking about other debates. The environment thus provides a kind of baseline case for thinking about "nature." In the course of further developing the account of "nature," the argument will seek to contribute to debates about how to go about protecting the natural environment. The chapter also criticizes a commonly accepted metaphysics of nature—a metaphysics that makes a sharp definition and a nonconstructivist account of nature compelling.

WILDERNESS: NATURE OR POST-NATURE

In environmental ethics, the question of how to understand what "nature" means is particularly crucial to two debates whose outcome would define the very objectives of environmentalism. The first is about the status of untouched, "pristine" nature—"wilderness." The impulse to preserve "pristine" nature is perhaps the very starting point of the environmentalist impulse. But is there any such thing any more? The second debate is about the status of *retouched* nature, as it were—environmental restoration. The loss of pristine nature has led many to try to recover nature by recreating it. But *can* there be any such thing as recreated nature? Some jettison the idea of pristine nature but readily accept the idea of environmental restoration; others put everything in the idea of untouched nature and are skeptical of environmental restoration. Both reject the idea that nature can be *restored*.

One of the earliest and most prominent critics of the concept of "nature" in environmental issues is the historian William Cronon, who, in 1995, started an influential essay with the sentence, "The time has come to rethink wilderness."[1] "The more one knows of its peculiar history," Cronon continued, "the more one realizes that wilderness is not quite what it seems." Reviewing that history, he argued that the concept of wilderness is an invented, constructed concept and, furthermore, that it has changed over time and frequently been wrong on the facts. In the United States, what is taken to be pristine nature is, in fact, often a product of thousands of years of human intervention. "Uninhabited wilderness" had included Indians and had typically been actively managed by them. "Wilderness" is not natural.

The problem with relying on this historically mistaken concept, Cronon explains, is that it leads to bad, irresponsible reactions to both social and environmental problems. Attending too much to wilderness can actually free us from attending seriously to the effect we have on the environment: "[T]o the extent that we live in an urban-industrial civilization but at the same time pretend to ourselves that our *real* home is in the wilderness, to just that extent we give ourselves permission to evade responsibility for the lives we actually lead."[2] It can lead us to try to protect rain forests in other countries (perhaps at the expense of poor peoples who live in those countries) rather than attending to environmental issues in our own communities and homes. It can lead us to avoid the kind of active management that may genuinely be needed to protect the environment. It can also lead us to accept social injustices, not only by preventing us from recognizing the claims that natives have to lands that we pretend they never inhabited but also simply by distracting us: if the preservation of wilderness is understood as a kind of metaphysical fight, then merely human moral problems can seem insignificant. On this point, Cronon quotes Earth First founder David Foreman as writing that the "preservation of wildness and native diversity is *the* most important issue. Issues directly affecting only humans pale in comparison."[3]

The fundamental mistake in the concept of wilderness, Cronon argues, is what he calls the "dualistic vision" of nature—the assumption that the human and the natural are distinct realms, each completely uncontaminated by the other. Cronon sees dualism about nature as a common but not inevitable mistake: "Wilderness gets us into trouble only if we imagine that this experience of wonder and otherness is limited to the remote corners of the planet, or that it somehow depends on pristine landscapes we ourselves do not inhabit."[4] "If wildness can stop being (just) out there and start being (also) in here, if it can start being as humane as it is natural, then perhaps we can get on with the unending task of struggling to live rightly in the world—not just in the garden, not just in the wilderness, but in the home that encompasses them both."[5] Thus Cronon formulates in an especially vivid and deeply felt way one of the central themes of this book: how to understand the separateness of nature.

For environmental philosopher Steven Vogel, dualism is an inevitable mistake with "nature." Vogel argues that the concept of nature is always the concept of *pristine* nature, nature untouched by humanity. Like Cronon, Vogel holds that pristine nature does not now exist, given the extent of human influence in the world. But Vogel goes beyond Cronon to hold that "nature," understood as pristine nature, can never be useful because it is never meaningful.

Vogel starts from Mill's dilemma: those who want to appeal to nature must say what the term refers to, and neither of the two most plausible definitions is useful—"nature" is either everything that accords with "the laws of nature," and humans cannot harm it, or it is everything other than what is human, and humans always and by definition harm it. Vogel sums up the damning dilemma this way:

> To be unhappy about the replacement of nature by a humanized world,...one must be able to point to some...empirical characteristic that the natural world possesses that a humanized one does not....That human beings can (but need not) destroy nature, that they can (but often do not) live in accordance with nature, that nature could (but often does not) serve as a normative model for their actions—these are all meaningful ideas, and yet if "nature" is being defined in the stipulative sense as that which is simply other than human action, then none of these ideas make much sense at all because they all either affirm or deny

(pointlessly, in either case) what the definition of nature analytically guarantees to be true.[6]

Vogel's target is the account exemplified by Eric Katz, who holds that "there is a fundamental ontological difference in the essential character of natural entities and human artifacts."[7] The difference is due to the role in their existence of human thought. "Artifacts exist only because of human intention and design. Artifacts are the physical manifestation of human purpose imposed on the world of nature."[8] But this explanation of the difference between artifact and nature amounts to a Cartesian dualism: "the mind is something other than the body; its products are different and somehow stand outside the world of nature. When *thought* is employed in the production of something, the product is thereby rendered 'artificial' and not natural."[9]

There is much to learn from and like about Descartes' metaphysics, but the basic idea that mind and body belong to distinct realms of being is not today much in favor, and to base environmentalism on it is to build a house on sand. Unfortunately, this is where any environmentalist position that understands nature as a realm untainted by human alteration necessarily ends because human alteration is always understood in terms of the imposition of intentionality.

What might an environmentalism that dispensed with pristine nature look like? Michael Pollan tries to work toward this kind of environmentalism in his book *Second Nature: A Gardener's Education*. Pollan, siding with Cronon, asks us to imagine an environmentalist ethos built around the concept of the *garden* rather than pristine nature or wilderness. The idea is meant as a compromise between the wilderness ethic and an ethic that cares nothing for nature. The gardener's ethic would be about "man *in* nature."[10] On the one hand, a gardener "doesn't spend a lot of time worrying about whether he has a god-given right to change nature."[11] A gardener's ethos would be "frankly anthropocentric." He would not be "romantic" about nature.[12] His overriding goal is to create places and produce things that are useful and pleasing. A gardener will merely work *with* nature: "The good gardener commonly borrows his methods, if not his goals, from nature herself.... It does seem that we do best in nature when we imitate her—when we learn to think like running water, or a carrot, an aphid, a pine forest, or a compost pile."[13] Instead of "pristine nature," then, Pollan recommends a "second nature"—a nature that is conceptually and causally connected both to nature and to human beings.

Chapter 1 argued that humans can be in "nature" simpliciter. Where "second nature" differs is in granting broader permission for the intentional

remaking of nature. A gardener's ethic is open to very different understandings of what the relationship of humans to nature aims at, and some
of these understandings seem openly at odds with what environmental
sentiment is all about. Pollan writes that "wilderness" is in reality a kind of
garden because it is "an indissoluble mixture of our culture and whatever it
is that's really out there."[14] By this standard, in which everything that mixes
human influence and the world outside human influence counts as "garden," not only is "wilderness" a kind of garden, so, too, is "open pit mine."
Pollan presumably wants to exclude the latter from consideration, but how?
And even if "open pit mine" is out, there would still be a huge range that
could count—and that for Pollan readily would count—as "garden." There
are gardens and gardens; some like what Pollan calls the Dionysian garden,
in which everything is rampant and wild and competing, the beans pulling
down the corn, the tomatoes shouldering out the beans, and the squash
spreading over the lawn, and others the Apollonian, in which everything is
kept in its row and weeds are eliminated each morning. Pollan holds that
humans are not just "in" nature but that the human role in nature is that
of master landscaper. We can discriminate among alternative plans according to what we find useful or pleasing. We can decide what kinds of scenes
and species we want. And, of course, some species might be pests and some
scenes eyesores. A gardener would be free to "try something completely
new," if it pleases his fancy.[15] Gardeners need not show forbearance. They
tire of an arrangement and rip it out. If a rare species does not happen to
contribute much to the artistic vision or utilitarian scheme that the gardener has in mind, then it is dispensable. Indeed, if artistic vision is the
guide, then the gardener probably *will* tire of the existing arrangements
and want something new, if only for the novelty; after all, art can be celebrated for being transgressive.

In short, a gardener's ethic might retain or entirely reject a preservationist impulse. Cronon notes that the concept of wilderness is present when
people speak of biodiversity and of the responsibility to protect endangered species; these, too, are ways of talking about the nonhuman part of
the world. Thus, to reject the wilderness ethic is apparently to deny that
there is particular value to nonhuman species. We might hope that a gardener will want to preserve nature in some measure, but that hope might
only replace a romantic idea of nature with a romantic idea of humans.

Cronon recognizes this problem, and he admits it makes him deeply
ambivalent about "wilderness." On the one hand, he writes, wilderness
is problematic because, under its influence, we are likely to see ourselves
as separate from nature. "On the other hand, I also think it no less crucial for us to recognize and honor nonhuman nature as a world we did not

create, a world with its own independent, nonhuman reasons for being as it is.... To the extent that wilderness has served as an important vehicle for articulating deep moral values regarding our obligations and responsibilities to the nonhuman world, I would not want to jettison the contributions it has made to our culture's ways of thinking about nature."[16]

Can we "rethink" wilderness, then? Can we make the concept of nature empirically meaningful, metaphysically sensible, and historically accurate, while also hanging onto the moral goal of preserving nature—of wanting to model the human relationship toward nature on an ideal of accommodating or preserving the natural world as we find it?

The idea introduced in Chapter 1 is that, in the contexts considered in this book, "nature" often has *something like* the second of Mill's definitions. Not always: if we are discussing the interactions among the species found in the Smokies and we note that some species, faced with new challenges, are doing what comes "naturally" and adapting to their new circumstances, then we are using "naturally" to refer to their innate capacities or maybe to the laws of nature (Mill's first sense) that make evolution possible. But if the conversation veers into a discussion of whether a species is present in the Smokies naturally or because of human interference, then we are operating with something like Mill's second sense of the term—something like "what is not human," implying independence from human affairs but not absolute independence. A thing can undergo some human alteration before we decide it is artifactual—recall John Passmore's account of environmental preservationism as "the attempt to maintain in their present condition such areas of the earth's surface as do not yet bear the *obvious* marks of man's handiwork."[17] What counts as "natural" shades gradually into what counts as "artifactual."

Moreover, Chapter 1 went on to propose that where that shading makes a decisive difference is a matter both of empirical fact and convention, as Passmore's use of the word "obvious" must suppose. "Obvious" here means *easily seen*, which requires reference to things that can be seen and to some seeing subject and to some account of what it is to see the relevant situation "easily." That a statement can be both factual and guided by convention is an easy point to understand in human contexts. Consider the sentence, "This brick structure is one of an assortment of buildings in the vicinity of Boston that were built in the nineteenth century to serve as Quaker meetinghouses." How many different layers of human convention are there in it? And yet it is plainly advancing a factual claim. Combining the ideas that a statement is guided both by the world and by human convention is tricky with "nature" because the relevant conventions are about what is independent of human interests, which seems to require that the rules for applying the concept must be independent of human convention. Worse, if "nature" is thought to mark a metaphysical distinction, then we may feel that the rules must have a timeless, eternal quality that feels incompatible with convention-dependence (and seems to require a sharp line of demarcation). But, in fact, nature may be said to be independent of us, even though the *concept* is very much dependent on us. (To ask that a concept be independent of human thought is really unfair.)

If the concept of "nature" is not explained as tracking a bright line running down the middle of the cosmos—a rabble of destructive humans on one side and pristine nature on the other—then it must be explained as relying on the very tools that Cronon brings to the fore. It must be understood historically rather than metaphysically. It must be *naturalized*—made a topic of empirical inquiry. To talk about whether a place is natural is to address the causal story that can be told about how the place came to be the way it is and the role of humans in that sequence. Historical analysis looks initially like a way of undoing claims about nature, but if we get clearer on what "nature" means (by allowing that the term is *not* clear), then historical analysis becomes a way of testing and refining those claims and undoing them only sometimes. Sometimes, we will realize that a widely accepted story turns out to be wrong, maybe even quite wrong, so that something we had thought "natural" begins to look artificial. And things can be "natural" to varying degrees, as Katz recognizes: "The human effect on the natural world is pervasive, but there are differences in human actions that make a descriptive difference. A toxic waste dump is different from a compost heap of organic material. To claim that both are equally non-natural would obscure important distinctions."[18] These are very good claims to make about "natural" and "artifactual" and the role of human action in determining whether something is one or the other, but they require that we have "descriptive" differences in mind—historical and empirical differences—rather than a metaphysical difference.

What kind of human causal role would be consistent with saying that a thing is natural? The sheer extent of human presence will be one consideration. A person standing alone in the forest, observing it and breathing the air, but not substantively altering it, would not render the scene "unnatural," but as a crowd gathers, and someone begins construction on a concession stand, the naturalness falters. It would be harder to experience a wilderness as part of a large tour group; the crowd would tend to hold the wilderness at bay. Another consideration will be whether humans have had a *central* role in the story of how the place came to be. This would square nicely with Katz's opposition, noted in Chapter 3, to human *domination* of nature. To rely on centrality is to further articulate the idea that nature is

that which is (more or less) independent of human causation. Yet centrality is very hard to sort out in causal stories. Suppose that bison evolved to
gather in vast herds as a defense against predation by humans; does that
make human activity "central" to the formation of those herds? Another
possible criterion is that a thing counts as natural when humans have not
greatly *damaged* it—by extinguishing the species existing in a place, for
example. This would mean that the critical issue is not simply the salience of
the human role, but its effects. It would square nicely with environmentalists' belief that it is sometimes possible for humans to help nature. Turning
a forgotten bit of prairie into a parking lot would make a place unnatural.
Carefully keeping out invasive species would not seem to. If destructiveness
is an important criterion, then not only does human presence not, by definition, make a thing unnatural, but human *management* would not necessarily make a thing unnatural. All of these ways of talking about how humans
affect the natural world are compatible with a preservationist impulse, but
they also all allow that humans can be in nature without nature thereby
becoming artifice. Probably, none of these ways are alone enough to fully
explain what it means for a place or a thing to be natural, however; some
of the general marks of nature that Kate Soper considers, and which were
mentioned in Chapter 1, point the way toward a still richer account.

This may seem to be a deflating position to reach about "nature."
Although it defends the main line of American environmentalist thought
insofar as it defends the idea of nature and makes possible a defense of the
preservationist impulse, it also departs from it by relinquishing the sharpest way of defining nature and the grandest way of declaring that it merits
preservation. We could still say, with John Muir, that nature is God's work,
but we cannot assert that God created nature as a metaphysically distinct
realm and that the metaphysical status of nature is the source of its moral
status—at least, we cannot say that if we want to be able to use the concept
of nature to make moral distinctions. And nature may seem to lose some
of its purity, not only because we no longer say that nature is absolutely
free of human involvement and because we admit that the idea of it is a
human construction. And, although we have found a way of understanding
"nature" that clears away some of the philosophical muddle and allows it
to make real distinctions, we have certainly not struck on a solution that
clears away all the factual muddle. In a debate about whether something is
natural, it will almost always be possible to call attention to some respect
in which the use of the term could be challenged. A given history can be
doubted, proven wrong, rewritten, and so on.

I think the conclusion is not deflating at all, though. First, it allows us to
retain the concept and to use it morally. Also, it allows that we *can* stand

in relationship to nature, for we deny that the only acceptable human relationship to nature is not to have anything to do with it. To say that nature admits human beings is simply to say that it is something we humans can touch. It is not a human impossibility, destroyed merely by breathing on it. To say that the concept of nature is a human concept admits a kind of anthropocentrism, but not one that should be troubling to environmentalists: It's one thing to say that our moral concepts are anthropocentric and another to say that our moral goals are anthropocentric. If we hold the preservation of "nature" as a value, we can indeed allow that the concept is anthropocentric—in the sense that it comes from us—while asserting that we humans are not the only things that we humans value.

RESTORATION: RETOUCHED NATURE

This more down-to-earth way of understanding the concept of nature also gives us a way of thinking about ecological restoration. If nature is understood as metaphysically distinct from what is humanly created, then to say that humans have "restored" a place to a natural state is to make a category mistake, and a particularly surprising and irritating one. This is Katz's view. "I am outraged," he writes, "by the idea that a technologically created 'nature' will be passed off as reality."[19] To say that a place has been restored to nature is to utter "The Big Lie," as he puts it. It is a conceptual impossibility because nature and artifacts are ontologically different—they are different at the level of *being*. Artifacts have an "inner nature or hidden essence" that is characterized by possession of an intrinsic purpose or function. This makes them "essentially anthropocentric. They are created for human use, human purpose—they serve a function for human life. Their existence is centered on human life."[20] Natural objects lack human purpose or function, and their existence is, as it were, their own.

Making naturalness dependent on the history of a thing rather than on its ontology makes possible a different and more complex account, I think. In the account of whether a natural thing can be made artifactual, various possible human roles were considered—such as that humans have come to have a central role in it and that humans have caused substantial harm to it. The goal of restoration, of course, is to try to correct, not merely limit, harm. Judged just by the standard of harm, a restored ecosystem is likely to count as "natural." The opposition to calling it natural is premised on the centrality of the human role. Suppose, for example, that an ecosystem that had been thoroughly destroyed were then recreated—from scratch, as it were. It would seem bizarre to call it natural. Creating a "natural" ecosystem from scratch does indeed sound like a conceptual impossibility. If there is a way to still call it natural, it is by noting that history is never completed. Suppose a thoroughly destroyed ecosystem has been immaculately restored, but the recreated biological and geological processes in it are then allowed to unspool on their own. At some point, it seems plausible to call it natural again. (If something becomes artifactual because human intentions have fundamentally changed its ontology, however, this gradual transition would be harder to make sense of; we would have to explain how a thing can gradually transition from one category of being to another.)

Many restoration efforts will fall somewhere in the middle: they will be corrections to damaged but not obliterated ecosystems, the restoration will require a lot of work but not a soup-to-nuts rebuilding, and the achievement will be well short of a complete recreation. In many of these cases, it will probably seem mistaken to say that nature has been restored—or, we will want to say it only while also immediately qualifying the claim and admitting that it can be challenged.

What makes Katz so irate about restoration is that if we admit restoration of nature is possible, then it looks like admitting that human ingenuity knows no bounds, that a technological fix is possible for any environmental problem, and therefore no one has any insurmountable reason to oppose any activity that causes environmental damage as long as the mess can be cleaned up later. Katz has surely got this right. We should agree up front that, just as a practical matter, human engineering can never fully recreate all the properties of a naturally occurring ecosystem. Proposing that human abilities will get to that point is a bit like proposing that if we knew everything about the state of the universe at a given time, then we could predict what a given person will be thinking a hundred years from now. Making the term "nature" dependent on claims about the history of a place can be responsive to Katz's concern, too: if a restored ecosystem is natural at all, it will not be unproblematically natural, whether we are thinking in terms of the harm done to nature or the centrality of the human causal role in recreating a place.

In short, we will end up with various and complicated things to say about whether a restored ecosystem is "natural." An absolute rejection of restoration would be implausible but so would an easy acceptance of it. In the Smokies, my impression is that restoration has mostly taken the form of dismantling the villages and homesteads that once stood there and allowing the forest to reclaim the land. (Whether I am right is a historical question, of course.) Not every human trace has been removed, however, and, of course, new roads and buildings have been constructed as well. Additionally, species have been reintroduced to the land, and measures have been taken to remove "non-native" species and protect threatened native species. Some of reintroduced species were actually closely related species—Western elk replaced Eastern elk, for example, which were not only gone from the Smokies but extinct throughout their range. What has been restored is now much closer to what was there, say, in 1800, but it is not identical. Is it "natural"? Is it "wilderness"? Under some senses often given to those words, they are misapplied if used to describe the Smokies. But, in comparison with many other places, describing it as natural seems defensible. If it is natural, of course, it is to some degree a "restored natural" place.

But now compare this situation with another, more radical restoration effort that some have proposed. "Pleistocene rewilding" is the effort to restore an ecosystem not merely to what it was like 200 years ago, but to its condition 10,000 or 15,000 years ago, by recreating the mix of species that has been missing since the extinction of the Pleistocene megafauna— mammoths, mastodons, ground sloths, glyptodonts, giant beavers, American lions, American cheetahs, saber-toothed tigers, dire wolves, and so on. The typical scenario proposed by proponents of Pleistocene rewilding is that similar species from other parts of the world would substitute for extinct species—African elephants for imperial mammoths, for example. This is obviously an imperfect solution because African elephants are adapted to particular food items and climates. Let's envision the ultimate technological fix, then, and imagine that the extinct species have been brought back to life by a clever mix of paleontology, DNA synthesis, and assisted reproduction. (The details are unimportant; human ingenuity knows no bounds, right?) Would a Smokies recreated in its Pleistocene image be "natural"?

I do not think so. Restoring the Smokies to roughly how it was 200 years is a kind of preservation, in the sense that it uncovers something there anyway, protects it in its original form, allows it, if Katz is right that it can exercise a kind of "autonomy," to carry on its history on its own terms. This kind of restoration is somewhat like restoring a piece of antique furniture by scraping away the recently applied green paint and replacing the new hinges with suitable old ones found at a scrapyard—hinges that are historically accurate and let the doors open in the way they're supposed to. But if restoration is a very radical overhaul, then it can no longer be described as a kind of preservation, and, at some point, even "restoration" will begin to feel inappropriate. It is instead more like a reenactment—a new creation modeled on something that is actually no longer in existence. If half the wood is replaced in our restored piece of furniture, then describing the work that has been done to it as "preservation" seems an unsustainable stretch. It has really been rebuilt. If all that remains is the upper right drawer, then the thing has not even been "rebuilt." A new piece of furniture has been built that incorporates an old drawer at the upper right. (Some episodes of "This Old House" come to mind.)

Given a sufficiently flexible understanding of "nature," we do not need to give up either preservationism or environmental restoration. Both can be understood as protecting a natural state of affairs. A further question, though, is whether we *may* protect nature, whether that is a legitimate use of state power.

A SPACE FOR NATURE

Wendell Berry responded to Thoreau's famous dictum, "In wildness is the preservation of the world" with the wry observation, "In human culture is the preservation of wildness."[21] To me, both epigrams seem right. Which is to say, one way Thoreau may have intended his dictum seems wrong. Thoreau may have meant to make a point about the location of truth and value—that these are grounded in something outside and beyond human affairs. Berry opposes this: truth and value are human claims and can be understood only in a human framework. But Thoreau's dictum can also be understood simply as a claim about the value of wildness (however that claim is thought to be grounded). Wildness is—or became, once the advance of human culture meant it was no longer an immutable fact of life—a deep human value. So understood, Berry offers not a retort, but advice: preserving wildness is a human business, and we should set out to do it. With *this*, Thoreau seems to have agreed, and some of his followers— John Muir and Muir's Sierra Club—have agreed passionately.

The question, then, is how to go about that business in a way that is consistent with the restrictions on policy in a liberal society. The four considerations in the preceding chapter offered a range of reasons for supposing, perhaps counterintuitively, that the liberal principle of neutrality concerning values that lie outside the overlapping consensus nonetheless requires some substantive engagement with them and support for them, that a hands-off policy stance toward them would be inadequate: (1) we do now, in an ostensibly liberal society, already go well beyond a hands-off stance; (2) some level of support for values outside the consensus is necessary if government is to pursue the basic goal of promoting human welfare; (3) since some of the other elements of a liberal society as we know it—namely, that it runs on a capitalist economy—tend to undermine some values, neutrality calls for evening the scale by offering those values some support; and (4) some level of support is necessitated by the moral value of respect for others, a value that lies at the very heart of liberalism.

How much support? When should or may government provide funding, and how much may it provide? When are constraints on individuals acceptable? When may government award people special rights (as it does to support marriage)?

These arguments imply not only that there can be a need for support, but also that there are built-in limits to that support. To engage with the particular intrinsic values that are caught up in different individuals' conceptions of human welfare, in order to promote their welfare, is to tolerate the variety of particular intrinsic values that are, in fact, present in a society; it provides no warrant for governmental endorsement of any of them nor for winnowing some of them out. To seek to redress the imbalances generated by a capitalist economy is only to aim at a better balance—again, not to endorse or eliminate any. And to show respect for others' intrinsic values by providing substantive support for them is very far from endorsing them and does not imply exclusion of others. The support offered is somewhat like that which an editor of a nonpartisan scholarly journal might offer to partisans: space for publication and help with articulating the message, but no assurance of winning the debate.

Public policy in the United States has so far moved to support the preservationist attitude (however imperfectly), but the support is undoubtedly limited, and government policy simultaneously supports a developmental stance. One of the interesting features of the preservationist ideal in the case of the environment is that the metaphor of "carving out space" can be put into practice in a nearly literal way: government can support that value by designating geographic space for it, through the creation of wildernesses, refuges, and national parks that exist side by side with national recreation areas, national forests, and reservoirs—spaces carved out for somewhat different purposes. The policy relies primarily on a comparatively modest form of coercion, that of taxation, although it has also included pressure brought to bear on the people initially living or working in these areas to move to other places or choose other lines of work or do their work in different ways (like catching fish or shrimp in ways that don't also snare dolphins or sea turtles). Funding can also be provided to give citizens incentives to protect animals or habitat (as mandated by the US Endangered Species Act).

Other policies are more coercive—zoning restrictions to limit development, limits or bans on hunting and fishing, bans on commercial trade of animals or animal parts, and so on. But are these policies so coercive as to amount to a kind of governmental endorsement of the preservationist stance? Not if there are other policies favoring development and limits or exemptions to the pro-preservationist policies. The underlying principle seems to be that there is some freedom of movement possible within a society. The activities that the law restricts can be taken elsewhere or practiced in a slightly different way; developers can turn to other parcels of land, hunters can hunt animals that are not endangered, "turtle excluder devices" do not exclude shrimping.

In short, the law tries to walk a line drawn between two poles. On the one hand, it seeks to provide genuine support for a preservationist value by creating and sustaining circumstances necessary for citizens to feel they are able to live by that value. This necessarily means that constraints are placed on other citizens; "carving out space" for one value means that space is restricted for another. But, on the other hand, it seeks to avoid constraints so powerful that they would amount to widespread forced allegiance to a value. It seeks to make it possible for people to hold alternative values.

Of course, only a little guidance is provided by pointing out that support for citizens' values is responsive to citizens' needs but limited by the need to balance values. A bit more substantive advice can be drawn out of the overall picture of how a liberal government is related to its citizens' moral values. That picture is a sort of complex Venn diagram. At the core is a circle delimiting values that government enforces. These are the "liberal" values. That humans are morally equal to each other is one of them. The periphery is a circle delimiting Rawls's "reasonable" values. A liberal government actively excludes judgments outside the circle. A judgment that some humans are worth less than others is one of those. Between the two circles are those values concerning which the liberal government aims ultimately at neutrality, seeking neither to endorse nor to exclude any, but potentially offering support. Now think of those values as themselves circles, with the size of the circle indicating the number of citizens who endorse the value and the distance the circle lies from the core values (the first large circle) indicating the strength of the arguments that support the value. (Of course, all this will be laughably or tear-jerkingly hard to judge of the actual moral views people have in the world, but so it always goes when we devise grand abstract principles to solve complex concrete problems.)

The size and distance of the reasonable but noncore values provide visual aids to illuminate two vague rules of thumb that a liberal government should follow. First, the case for supporting a value is greater when more people endorse a value—when the circle is bigger. In other words, the decision concerning which values to support and how much support to offer should factor in the representation of that value in the citizenry. This amounts to something less than majoritarianism, since government should also still try to avoid compelling allegiance to a value, but it reflects what makes majoritarianism attractive.

It is the second and third arguments for government support that suggest this majoritarian element. If a very large portion of the population finds great value in the natural world, government will more effectively advance the general welfare by promoting that value, and, indeed, it could be hard to advance the general welfare while avoiding that value. The policy implications of respect for others' values also seem to be sensitive to size. If respect for others entails some level of support for their value positions, then, if very many people share a particular value position, the argument that society ought to support it seems greater. Our school system in a village in Westchester County, New York, closes for the Jewish holidays; the schools I attended growing up in a small town in Tennessee did not. Possibly, given the very different demographics of the two communities, both decisions make sense. One of the reasons environmental preservationism has led to policy, then, is that it enjoys fairly broad support among the public.

The case for social support is also likely to be stronger, more easily made, when the value is relatively accessible to reasonable citizens—when the value is comparatively easy to understand, when it is fairly easy to become a participant in that value oneself, when participating in it does not withdraw one from society into a distinct secondary society. The core moral values are the most accessible, of course. In fact, we expect that people not only *can* share them; we expect that they do. Moral discussions at this level often proceed by simply describing facts or enumerating the values, in hopes that the interlocutor will come along with us and see things as we do: why shouldn't your friend treat her neighbor that way? Because it's cruel. ("Surely you see that! What's wrong with you?") Very likely, no deeper justification is expected or even possible. The question, "But what's wrong with treating people cruelly?" would most likely elicit incredulity.

Many other values are not universally shared but are still comparatively accessible. Many of the values in sports are like this. Here, too, moral discussions tend to be about both facts and values. If a sports fan were asked why he cares about sports, for example, he is likely simply to talk about the games, the players, his feelings about them—he is likely to say things, that is, that are aimed at engendering a similar emotional reaction from the listener, in hopes that the listener will feel the value from the inside. Certainly, not everyone cares about sports, but it is not a big leap to become someone who does. There is no particular social line between those who do and those who do not. At the further end are values that are less easily accepted, whose justification requires reference to a larger worldview or to a particular metaphysics, and acceptance of which draws one into a new community: "Why should primary school education be more Bible-based? Because it is important that children be brought up within a Christian belief system, which we know to be true on the basis of our faith."

People argue for environmental preservation in both metaphysically accessible and metaphysically arcane ways. Thoreau himself worked on different levels at once, occasionally down to earth and occasionally religious or quasi-religious. When he wrote, "In wildness is the preservation of the world," for example, he probably meant in part to refer to Nature (capitalized) as a realm that is never known more than partially, that always opens up to new lines of understanding, both of the world and of ourselves, and therefore provides, as Robert Dorman has written, interpreting Thoreau, "an unlimited setting for novel experience—for *freedom*."[22] Nature was also the source of what is truly good and beautiful, whereas civilization was, often at least, characterized by meanness. Because the pursuit of what is good and beautiful would therefore mean a rejection of "the tyranny of public opinion," freedom meant self-expression and self-realization and the "Life Without Principle," as Thoreau put it in the title of an essay. Thus, Wildness and, by extension, Nature were also fundamentally subversive concepts. Indeed, Nature could be anarchic; by always surpassing human understanding and human concepts it could open up to a kind of meaninglessness: this is the force of Thoreau's musings about the Nature he experienced atop Mt. Ktaadin:

This was that Earth out of Chaos and Old Night. Here was no man's garden, but the unhandseled globe. It was not lawn, nor pasture, nor mead, nor woodland, nor lea, nor arable, nor waste land. It was the fresh and natural surface of the planet Earth, as it was made forever and ever. . . . There was clearly felt the presence of a force not bound to be kind to man. . . . Talk of mysteries! Think of our life in nature,—daily to be shown matter, to come in contact with it,—rocks, trees, wind on our cheeks! the *solid* earth! the *actual* world! the *common sense*! *Contact! Contact! Who* are we? *Where* are we?[23]

At other times, Nature seemed to Thoreau more benevolent, although still surpassing human understanding. In these moods, Thoreau was apt to speak of Nature as a kind of personality: "It is as if I always met in those places [in the Maine wilderness] some grand, serene, immortal, infinite, encouraging, though invisible companion, and walked with him."[24] In all of this—as a field of human freedom, as a subversive prod to a deeper moral understanding, as a transcendent force or personality—Nature was the seat of the divine, and it was by contact with Nature that one could be conscious of the divine.

But Thoreau could also write of nature in a simpler, down-to-earth vein, as a realm of ponds and birds and animals and thawing ice and trees. And he did, recording detailed observations in thousands of pages of notes and tables. An entire chapter of *Walden* is built around a discussion of the pond's winter ice. This aspect of Thoreau—this simpler sense of wonder in and appreciation of nature—is to some degree severable from Thoreau's claims about the divinity present in nature, for although Thoreau himself might, if pressed, have traced that sense of wonder back to its philosophical roots, readers are able to understand and appreciate the sense of wonder without drawing on that background. And this aspect of Thoreau has descendants in Muir, who also moved back and forth between secular writing about nature and claims that nature embodies and reveals religious truths, and Leopold, who grounded his environmental ethics in accounts of his experiences in nature.

Insofar as we agree with Berry that the preservation of wildness depends on culture, it is this simpler, grounded account of nature—nature naturalized, rather than nature as the seat of the divine—that we must have in mind. Culture will not preserve the divinity that Thoreau found in nature; by Thoreau's lights, it threatens the death of *that*. But it is certainly human culture that can best preserve ponds, birds, animals, and trees from human encroachment.

Perhaps the capacity to value nature is not entirely severable from some religious perspective. To the extent that it is not, there is added reason for some caution about promoting it through the exercise of governmental powers. Leopold, however, is a pivotal figure in environmental ethics partly because he brings the justification down to the level of descriptions and patterns of reaction; he does not turn to underlying metaphysical claims but instead asserts rather baldly that nature has moral value (indeed, in Leopold's view, standing in the community of moral beings). Leopold's writing is philosophical in the sense of being reflective and sensitive, but it contains little that would count as reasoned argument or justification for his position by the standards of analytic philosophy. I argued in Chapter 2, however, that the role of argument in morality is *within* morality, rather than to give it foundations. This philosophical framework makes sense of Leopold's method by giving up on the possibility of ultimate justification and pointing up the importance of the kind of descriptions that Leopold gives us, which serve to evince and elicit the right moral reactions. Since Leopold, it has been possible to speak of the value of nature without adverting to underlying religious or metaphysical claims about nature.

Because environmental preservationism is reasonably widely shared and reasonably accessible, government support for it is reasonable. Moreover, although any government support for it will be coercive to some degree, government support for environmental preservationism need not be maximally coercive: it is possible to set aside some places and protect some species and ecological systems without, in effect, demanding that citizens honor environmental preservationism throughout their lives. They can, as it were, relocate themselves within society. None of this makes policy decisions about environmental preservationism easy. But it offers the possibility of successfully walking the line between supporting those citizens for whom environmental preservationism is important without excluding competing perspectives.

The other way to pursue some of the goals of the preservationist attitude, of course, is to find aid in the more central and broadly endorsed goal of promoting the common weal. Nature must be protected to protect public health, refresh resources important to economic growth, provide a ground for medical and industrial discovery, widen the possibilities for recreation, create beautiful spaces, and so on. If the argument in Chapter 4 is correct, some of these overtly welfarist goals themselves subtly cross-reference various less central and specialized values, but, given that there is something of a spectrum from relatively utilitarian conceptions of welfare to conceptions that are bound up intimately with richer values, there is still some point in holding that appeals to the common weal are *more* central. And some preservationist goals, such as trying to limit global warming and ocean acidification, are also hugely important for comparatively straightforward utilitarian reasons. But it will be obvious to most environmentalists that the common weal language will not achieve everything a preservationist wants. For one thing, the language will not support some preservationist goals nearly so well—preserving relatively unvisited "wilderness" areas and endangered species, for example. For another, some strategies for combatting global warming will themselves be intrinsically unattractive to a preservationist. Some of the "geoengineering" proposals—for banks of sunblocking mirrors in orbit around the earth, for example, or for reflective aerosols distributed in the atmosphere—are disheartening even if they might actually work.

NOTES

1. William Cronon, "The Trouble with Wilderness; Or, Getting Back to the Wrong Nature," in *Uncommon Ground: Rethinking the Human Place in Nature*, ed. William Cronon (New York: W. W. Norton and Co., 1995), 69–90, at 69.
2. Ibid., 82.
3. Ibid., 84.

4. Ibid., 88.

5. Ibid., 90.

6. Steven Vogel, "Why 'Nature' Has No Place in Environmental Philosophy," in *The Ideal of Nature: Debates about Biotechnology and the Environment*, ed. Gregory E. Kaebnick (Baltimore, Md.: Johns Hopkins University Press, 2011), 84–97, at 89–90.

7. Eric Katz, "Preserving the Distinction Between Nature and Artifact," in *The Ideal of Nature: Debates about Biotechnology and the Environment*, ed. Gregory E. Kaebnick (Baltimore, Md.: Johns Hopkins University Press, 2011), 71–83, at 73.

8. Ibid.

9. Vogel, "Why 'Nature' Has No Place in Environmental Philosophy," 93.

10. Michael Pollan, *Second Nature: A Gardener's Education* (New York: Grove Press, 1991), 190.

11. Ibid., 191.

12. Ibid. 192.

13. Ibid., 194–95.

14. Ibid., 191.

15. Ibid., 195.

16. Cronon, "The Trouble with Wilderness," 87.

17. John Passmore, *Man's Responsibility for Nature: Ecological Problems and Western Traditions* (New York: Charles Scriber & Sons, 1974), 101, italics added.

18. Eric Katz, *Nature as Subject: Human Obligation and Natural Community* (Lanham, Md.: Rowman & Littlefield, 1997), 104.

19. Ibid., 97.

20. Ibid., 98.

21. Wendell Berry, "Getting Along with Nature," in *Home Economics* (San Francisco, Cal.: Northpoint Press, 1987), 11.

22. Robert Dorman, *A Word for Nature: Four Pioneering Environmental Advocates, 1845–1913* (Chapel Hill: University of North Carolina Press, 1998), 77. The following paragraphs draw heavily on Dorman's account of Thoreau.

23. Henry David Thoreau, "The Maine Woods" (New York: Thomas Y. Crowell & Company, 1909), 92–93.

24. Quoted in Dorman, *A Word for Nature,* 63.

CHAPTER 6

Nature on the Farm

Genetically Modified Plants and Animals

The genetic modification of plants and animals has been one of the flash points in moral arguments about nature in recent decades. What the objection is, though, is as hard to express as it is deeply felt. It is rarely articulated clearly. As the agricultural ethicist Paul Thompson has pointed out, critics tend to make their case "more through innuendo than through direct statement."[1] Sometimes, the case is made with angry labels. Critics call food that contains genetically modified (GM) organisms "Frankenfood," and they call the Monsanto Company, leading developer of GM crops, "Monsatan." Often, Thompson notes, the argument consists of incredulous questions: "What is wrong with a cow the size of an elephant, or a sheep the size of a horse, or 'glowing' tobacco plants? Is there any meaning in the morphology of animals and plants...?"[2] When a genetically modified fluorescent zebrafish was introduced, a California Fish and Game commissioner explained his vote to forbid sale of the fish in California with this comment: "For me, this is a question of values, not a question of science.... I look at this and ask myself, 'So what's next? Pigs with wings? Pink horses?'"[3] Prince Charles once registered his opposition to GM organisms by writing that biotechnology has "brought us to a crossroads of fundamental importance. Are we going to allow the industrialisation of Life itself?"[4]

Even sophisticated scholarly defenses of this feeling tend to rely on questions designed to elicit intuitions. A group of European ethicists led by Bernice Bovenkerk concluded that the philosophical case against GM animals needs work but also that the position deserves a careful hearing in spite of its problems because the intuitions are pretty clear. Consider a proposed genetic modification to egg-laying chickens: currently, these chickens are forced to endure intolerable living conditions, but perhaps genetic technologies offer a solution. "What if we could make these animals adjust better to their environment and genetically engineer them into senseless humps of flesh, solely directed at transforming grain and water into eggs?"[5] The chicken-flesh humps would be "living egg machines"—valuable industrial tools and, being tools, incapable of being harmed.

The wider public has not come down firmly against GM organisms, but it has misgivings. Surveys have reliably shown that a significant portion of the public finds GM organisms morally troubling. A 2004 study by the Food Policy Institute at Rutgers University found that sizable minorities disapprove of genetically engineered food and especially of food from genetically engineered animals.[6] In a 2005 poll conducted by the Pew Initiative on Food Biotechnology, two-thirds of respondents said they were "uncomfortable" about animal cloning even though less than half thought the products were unsafe.[7] A market research firm hired by a company that clones livestock reported that more than a third of those it polled said they would not buy such products even when first told that the US Food and Drug Administration (FDA) was likely to declare them safe.[8] Three-quarters of respondents to a poll paid for by the International Food Information Council said that they had an unfavorable impression of animal cloning.[9] Disapproval of genetically modified food is stronger in Europe; in a 2001 study using focus groups from five countries, participants said they wanted GM foods labeled, and *"not simply in order to be able to protect themselves against putative health risks*. Labeling was also felt to be important to allow consumers to boycott the products in order [to] 'send a message' to manufacturers about a whole range of concerns other than health risks."[10]

Scholarly opinion is divided between those like Bovenkerk and colleagues, struggling to articulate the philosophical case against living egg machines, and those like Thompson, who points out that the absence of a clear case is cause for doubt. Those "who would turn inchoate concern into a strong prohibition of genetic engineering," writes Thompson, should "attempt an explicit statement of such an argument, if only to clarify and sharpen the terms of debate."[11] Some prominent scholarly analyses reject the case as incoherent from the outset. The idea that "there are certain things humans were not meant to do . . . is certainly operative regarding genetic engineering of animals," acknowledges the agricultural ethicist Bernard Rollin. "Some theme such as this is often orchestrated in tabloid accounts of genetic engineering—the key notion is that there is something intrinsically wrong with genetic engineering: blurring species, 'messing with nature,' violating the sanctity of life, 'playing god,' and so forth."[12] Rollin concludes that these claims mostly "involve religious appeals that cannot be translated into secular moral terms, appeals to portentous and vacuous notions ..., and appeals to questionable metaphysical categories."[13] Those that don't turn out to be questions about harm to animals, Rollin concludes—not questions about the intrinsic wrongness of genetic modification.

Thus, the debate about how agricultural biotechnology intersects with values concerning the human relationship to nature has become a sharply delineated, either-or contest. Some suggest that agricultural biotechnology is heinous and abominable, that it violates something sacred. Others are entirely dismissive.

Can we speak of what is "natural" in agriculture? The concept of nature— of the world independent of human intervention—is baffling enough when we are talking about the natural environment. But the environment is the easy case; it is easy to see how "wildernesses" could be entirely independent of human intervention (even if the tracts of land described as wildernesses turn out, in fact, to have been shaped by people). In agriculture, to speak of nature is—apparently—to propose that something which is all about human intervention could, at the same time, be independent of human intervention. Can we meaningfully talk at all of a "natural" way of growing corn, for example, given that the plant we know as corn has, through several millennia of human selection, changed enough that it took some scientific sleuthing just to identify its ancient forebear?

In general, the domesticated forms of plants are dramatically different from their wild forebears, in appearance, growth habit, and taste. Sometimes the wild form of an edible and nutritious plant is unpalatable, even toxic. And then planting, cultivating, and harvesting are human activities, all ways of initiating, managing, or halting nature's processes. Domesticated animals, too, have undergone an assortment of changes from their wild forebears—cows are said to bear no more than a very strong resemblance to the Eurasian aurochs from which they are descended—and breeding, raising, and slaughtering them are all matters of human agency. "Nature abhors a garden," concludes Michael Pollan,[14] and She probably resents ranches.

Agricultural biotechnology is an important case study for thinking about the human relationship to nature both because it is a domain in which concerns about that relationship are prominent and because it involves some special complexities in the account so far developed of those appeals. In particular, it gives an opportunity to think further about how to identify "nature" and how to develop policy that "carves out a space" for the value some give to nature.

WHAT'S GROWING

A brief overview of the history of GM organisms will illustrate just what sort of challenge they present to the human relationship to nature and set that challenge in the context of the larger moral debate about their use. The history is somewhat mixed, as some GM organisms have been market failures. The first GM crop to hit the market—the "Flavr Savr" tomato, engineered to ripen on the vine yet remain firm and durable during transport to market—was pulled in 1997 when it failed to catch on with consumers, and Monsanto pulled its "NewLeaf" GM potatoes shortly after McDonald's announced that it would buy only nonmodified potatoes. Another noteworthy failure was an experimental tomato that, thanks to a gene from an arctic flounder, was supposed to be frost-resistant and capable of withstanding cold storage. The "fish tomatoes," as some critics called them, were ultimately not successful, the effort was abandoned, and the company, DNA Plant Technology, went out of business.

Many other GM crops have become a major part of modern agriculture in many parts of the world, however. Data from the US Department of Agriculture (USDA) indicates that in 2012, roughly 90 percent of all soybeans, cotton, and corn grown in the United States was genetically modified.[15] The modifications to these plants are all of two sorts: they have been given herbicide tolerance, on the grounds that they allow farmers to eliminate weeds by spraying even after the crop has germinated, or they have been made to produce a pesticide themselves, in theory freeing farmers from having to spray or dust.

An assortment of other GM crops have also been approved and worked their way into the market, sometimes in fits and starts. Genetically modified alfalfa, for example, which had been made to tolerate herbicide, was approved for planting, then banned by court order, then reapproved.[16] Other kinds of modifications have been developed but not yet approved, including crops designed to have superior growth characteristics— drought-resistance, for example—and to produce foods with better nutritional qualities.[17]

In general, concluded a 2010 report from the National Research Council, GM crops have had "substantial net environmental and economic benefits to U.S. farmers" when compared against conventional crops.[18] They have led to reduced pesticide use, to the use of less toxic pesticides, and to a more flexible schedule for applying pesticides, for example. The opponents of GM crops raise concerns primarily about the long-term, unanticipated consequences of the GM revolution. One of the most common genetic modifications causes plants to produce a protein that, in the wild, is produced by a soil-dwelling bacterium called *Bacillus thuringiensis* (Bt), which is itself considered a pesticide, highly effective yet milder than many alternatives, and is commonly used in organic farming. Critics of GM crops have argued that engineering entire crops to produce the insect-killing protein in *B. thuringiensis* will tend to speed the evolution of insects that tolerate it, so that, in the end, what looks like a valuable new agricultural technique might actually *deprive* farmers of one.[19] (Planting small plots of non-Bt crops alongside fields of Bt crops seems to work pretty well in short-circuiting the emergence of resistance: insects that lack resistance to Bt can survive in these plots, insects with resistance can then mate with them, and the alleles that provide resistance are then less likely to become predominant in the insect population. Farmers often ignore this advice, however.)

The best case for GM foods is perhaps "golden rice." Rice plants normally produce beta carotene in all parts of the plant except for the endosperm, but golden rice plants produce it in the endosperm as well, giving the rice a golden hue. The genetic manipulation is not very dramatic compared to the "fish tomato" and perhaps it is a less violent-seeming intrusion into nature. Moreover, golden rice was developed as a way of improving nutrition in developing countries, it was developed by academic researchers rather than by profit-seeking private enterprises, and the researchers plan to have it freely distributed to farmers in developing countries.

The GM animals that have so far been developed have been given disparate properties. "Heart-healthy" pigs have been engineered that, thanks to roundworm genes, produce omega-3 fatty acids in their flesh, raising the prospect of buying bacon that's good for you. The Enviropig has been engineered to excrete less phosphorus in its manure, making these pigs' manure less environmentally damaging. Neither pig has made it to market. The AquAdvantage salmon is likely to be the first GM animal approved for consumption in the United States; by early 2013, anyway, it still appeared to be working its way slowly through the FDA's approval process. This salmon has received one gene (from another kind of salmon) for producing growth hormone and a genetic switch (from another fish, the ocean pout) that keeps the salmon growing in cold weather, when normally its growth would pause. The salmon does not grow bigger than an unmodified salmon, but it grows twice as fast, reaching market size in one and a half years instead of three years.[20] According to AquaBounty Technologies, the company developing the fish, the salmon requires less feed and care to reach full size, which makes it environmentally beneficial.

The only genetically engineered animal yet to reach the market in the United States is the Glofish—the fluorescent zebrafish mentioned earlier.

Developed by Yorktown Technologies as a tool for detecting pollution (the idea was that the fish would glow only in the presence of certain pollutants), the fish has instead been sold primarily as a pet.[21]

As several of these examples illustrate, genetic modification could, in principle, serve various goals in agriculture. It could be used to produce better foods or to produce foods in better ways. In practice, it has mostly been used to improve farming efficiency. It is a way of extending the Green Revolution—the development of high-yield varieties of plants and new strategies for growing them. The latter include irrigation systems and fertilizers, pesticides, and herbicides to drive growth and curtail things that limit growth. The new varieties succeed in part because they channel their energies into seed or fruit rather than, say, roots or stems. This means, though, that they are high-maintenance plants: they are more dependent on irrigation, pesticides, and herbicides. Some of them (corn, for example) have also been specially bred to tolerate high-density planting, increasing yields still further. All of these factors together encourage mechanization, and mechanization in turn requires monoculture agriculture—growth of vast swaths of a single variety that can be planted, watered, dosed, and harvested simultaneously by machines. GM plants (at least those so far put into use) contribute to this overall strategy by taking over some of the pesticide dosing or lending themselves to heavier herbicide dosing. They are designed, in short, for monoculture. It is no surprise, then, that the vast majority of them are grown on large industrial farms.[22]

QUESTIONS ABOUT GM ORGANISMS: HARM TO ANIMALS

What is it about certain ways of relating to species on the farm that is troubling for some people? In particular, what is wrong with the genetic modification of organisms? One straightforward position—a detour from the concern that genetic modification is an intrinsically objectionable relationship to nature, but possibly a surrogate for that less easily articulated position—is that it's likely to be harmful to the animals. Certain things we do to animals in agricultural settings simply cause them to have worse lives. Feeding corn to beef cows to fatten them up for the market makes their stomachs bloat, for example, because cows' stomachs are not well evolved to process corn. Belgian Blue cattle, bred to exploit a naturally occurring mutation for "double-muscling," are unable to give birth naturally. Conceivably, permitting the genetic modification of animals could take this tendency to another level.

Genetic modification is often premised on the thought that genes work in a fairly simple way: they provide instructions for the body, and they typically provide instructions to do some particular thing. Thus, the causal connections are one-directional (from genes to the body) and one-to-one (a given gene codes for a given trait). The latter idea, called the *central dogma*, is now widely abandoned; in fact, a given gene can have different effects in different parts of the body, or at different points in development, or when the organism grows in a different environment. The former, found in the idea that the genetic code is the Book of Life, is accepted as a truism by many biologists but has been rejected by others. Systems biologists, for example, argue that there are various feedback mechanisms within the body that affect genetic expression. The causal connections form a loop, or even a set of loops, such that no one part can be described as the one controlling part.[23]

Given these complications, the effects of a given genetic modification are much harder to understand and predict than has typically been acknowledged. A given genetic change could turn out to do something unexpected and unwanted, or it could lead to changes in other bodily mechanisms as the body tries to accommodate it. Making genetic changes is a complicated business, and the outcome of a genetic change is harder to predict than one might like. The example of "living egg machines" establishes that the *goal* of genetic engineering might be beneficent; the worry is that such goals would prove unattainable and that the actual practice would tend to go awry.

Concerns about harm are not decisive. In fact, it is conceivable that genetic modifications will prove beneficial to animals. In theory, we could end up designing GM animals that are better suited to life on the farm, eat GM plants that are better suited for their needs, and are outfitted with GM gut microbes that let them better digest those plants. Perhaps GM animals would have brains and personalities perfectly suited to industrial animal husbandry, if industrial animal husbandry is not an oxymoron. Or, possibly, things will not go so well, and animals would be better off if we focused on improving husbandry and shifting away from the industrial approach to it. Questions about how use of the technology might actually turn out are important regardless of how we respond morally to the very idea of modifying them, of course.

SPECIES INTEGRITY

The most common way of defending the intrinsic objection to GM agriculture is to argue that it violates organismic integrity. Starting with the premise that life in general has value, the environmental philosopher Holmes Rolston III argues that "Organisms are normative systems." A plant, for example, "is a spontaneous life system, self-maintaining with a controlling program.... It executes this project, checking against performance in the world. It composes and recomposes itself, maintaining order against disordering tendencies." A plant has *integrity*. Animals, too, have integrity, but one raised to another level through their subjectivity: "there is something here behind the fur and feathers. They have eyes. The animal life, with its centered experience, is organic form in locomotion."[24] Strictly, the integrity of organic form is something that characterizes *species*, in Rolston's account, although it is instantiated in individuals: "The integrity sought, the value defended, is an ideal toward which a wild life is striving. In the language of the geneticists, the integrity lies in that phenotype produceable by the normal genotype in a congenial environment."[25] "When genotype develops into phenotype, presumptively at least each species, instantiated in individuals, is a worthwhile biological achievement and an adapted fit in its niche. Each is a distributed increment of [generic] life on Earth, instancing the richness of life collectively on this marvelous planet."[26]

I have never been confident that I have quite grasped the logical structure of this position, but I think the core argument goes like this: life is widely thought to have value, and to value life means to value species because species are the forms that life actually takes in the world. To value life also means to value integrity—the property of maintaining order against disordering forces—because integrity is the fundamental characteristic of life and because it is impossible to value any species without valuing its unique way of maintaining order. And to value life means to value individual organisms because, although "the type is more important than the token,"[27] still, the token is the concrete instantiation of the species and so it is through our treatment of the token that we can value the type.

The primary problem with the argument is that it tries to show that genetic modification conflicts with values found in nature herself (this is a gambit for objectivity, as I argued in Chapter 2), yet, as many have noted, nature in fact seems to have little interest in maintaining genetic order. Species, as we know them in the world, are not fixed. They evolve, themselves "recomposing" spontaneously into new forms. Nor, at any one time, are species always clearly delineable; biologists sometimes disagree about whether a group of animals belongs to a single species or falls into different although very similar species (or "subspecies," further complicating the situation). Nor do species themselves appear to respect species boundaries. Animals occasionally interbreed; wolves and coyotes are agreed to be distinct species, but the coyotes now found in the Eastern United States may be the result of some wolf–coyote pairing (and are thus perhaps not quite the same species as Western coyotes). Moreover, humans have at times interbred species—mating horses with donkeys to produce mules, for example—and the process has not generally been decried. Genetic modification would introduce further variation, but the basic idea of stirring the genetic pot is not new.

A further complication has to do with the way Rolston talks about species and the individual organisms that belong to them. Rolston points out that the integrity that purportedly characterizes a species is actually an *ideal*—meaning here an unrealized goal—toward which wild life—a species as we know it in the world—is only striving. Rolston is directing our attention at this point toward an ancient metaphysical philosophical debate about types, tokens, and their reality. The nominalist position is that types—kinds—are mere constructions and that what actually exists are only individuals. The realist position, which Rolston endorses, is that kinds, although abstract, have a reality that transcends the reality of individuals; the individuals concretely instantiate the kind but are also ephemeral and imperfect. The integrity of the kind endures even when individuals depart from its perfection; indeed, even when individuals are absent altogether.

But now the problem with basing the argument against genetic modification on species integrity is the opposite of the one presented earlier: species—kinds—are so very changeless and permanent that they cannot be damaged by anything done to concrete instantiations of them. "[N]one of it matters to the species at all," notes Bernard Rollin, "for things do not matter to species, and, if one is a realist, species continue to exist whether or not their members do!"[28] What is needed, in order to show that genetic modification is wrong, are some further premises. First, we must stipulate that the abstractions that are the ultimate reality provide a moral guide to the creatures who populate the imperfect physical world; this would make it wrong to modify creatures so that they depart from the species-typical abstractions. Also, to work specifically against genetic modifications achieved technologically while permitting conventional agricultural practices (breeding or environmental change) that cause members of a species to depart from the species norm, we must assert that the true nature of a species—its essence—is encoded in the genes. If genes are metaphysically different, then modifications to them can be especially objectionable.

These claims about kinds, essences, and the special metaphysical status of genes are the "questionable metaphysical categories" Rollins complains about. There are smart people who accept these claims; they are not patently nonsensical. But they are something of a stretch for many others; they would certainly require some very special defense. The idea that modifying an organism's genes is tantamount to changing its essence is particularly problematic; the assumption seems to be that genes are a special link connecting the physical and the metaphysical—a modern version of Descartes' claim that the pineal gland was the seat of the soul, the spot in the body that connected the body with the mind. The mere fact that genes from different species, even different kingdoms, can be combined in an organism to produce surprising results (sometimes so surprising that even the researchers do not expect them) itself seems to cast doubt on the idea that the genes provide access to the essence of an organism. That idea also does not comport well with the view that genes do not work as one-directional instructions to the body, that their function is controlled by the body. The "essence" of an organism—to the extent that we can speak of it—is something that has to do with *all* parts of the body. The genes obviously play a very significant role within the body, and modifying them is a good way of trying to change the body, but if we are concerned about the alteration of nature, we should pay special attention to the genes only because and to the extent that they offer one effective way of making alterations. There is nothing magical about them. If we are concerned about the human modification of other species' nature, then every kind of modification is on the table.

PURITY

The difficulty of using "nature" clearly in the agricultural context has, of course, not gotten in the way of using it frequently. Some of these uses are not much more than mere marketing pap, however. The worst are the grandest and most sweeping, such as that a food product is "all natural," "100 percent natural," or "made from 100 percent natural ingredients." These statements contrast "natural" with "artificial" or manufactured and sometimes also suggest that "natural" foods are free of chemicals. The core idea, I believe, is that natural foods have a kind of purity: there is no human stain on them.

In any of these ways of understanding "natural," of course, all foods are unnatural. All food items purchased in stores have been processed, and sometimes what is sold as "natural" is very heavily processed. Sometimes, too, the processing could even be described as preserving "naturalness": frozen vegetables sometimes preserve more of the plant's naturally occurring vitamins than do "fresh" vegetables. Likewise, all foods are composed of chemicals, and they are healthful (or toxic) only in virtue of the chemicals they contain. Many foods even include an assortment of chemical or bio-logical agents—colorings or other ingredients—yet may still qualify as "natural." Colored, fried vegetable chips may count as natural, for example, if the coloring and the frying oil are extracted from plants through appro-priate processes.

Plainly, even if the problems that afflict the concept of "nature" in the environmental context had not already convinced us, defining "natural" as meaning "free of human intervention" will not work. "Free of chemicals" is a complete nonstarter, and "free of human stain," remembering the dis-cussion of nature in the environmental context, is little better. The envi-ronmental context also suggests, however, that we could find a way to peg "natural" to the degree or kind of human involvement rather than to the mere fact of human involvement. If a food is processed *too much,* or in too dramatic a fashion, we might still say, as a matter of convention, that the alteration is "unnatural."

In the use of "nature" in debates about the environment, what under-writes acceptance of a rougher definition—one only approximating Mill's second sense of the term—is our ability to elucidate "natural" in terms of the human and nonhuman causal contributions. This parsing can get some traction in the environmental case because we genuinely can point to non-human elements of the story, and we can talk about whether the human role is "central" or "dominating" in our telling of how the scenario in front of us (Kate Soper's "lay concept" of nature) came to be. There is a full spec-trum of cases of "natural," even if those all the way over on the "natural" end are now only the landscapes of distant planets and prehistoric times. This spectrum allows us to group contemporary landscapes toward one or the other end depending on the history of the place. So, we can say that a parking lot is artificial and a given patch of forest in the Smoky Mountains count as "natural."

The case of agriculture forces us to press this sort of reasoning a little further. In agriculture, the human role is perhaps so thorough, so central to the very idea of "cultivating" plants and "domesticating" animals, that perhaps the term "natural" is never really plausible.

A CONVERSATION WITH NATURE

I have presented concerns about human alteration of the environment as a kind of base case for thinking morally about human modification of other naturally occurring phenomena, such as the nature of humans and other species. Moral concerns about the modification of other species would have to be articulated a little differently from concerns about *preserving* the environment: agricultural species are already so heavily modified, and ongoing modification of nature is already so widely accepted—breeding, seeding, weeding—that we cannot meaningfully talk of *preservation*. In explaining environmentalism, we relinquished a purist sense of nature and allowed that human-influenced places might still count as "natural," but, in agriculture, that way of speaking is too stretched to really be applicable. In short, the case for talking about "a human relationship to nature" seems rather weak when we think about nature in the context of agriculture. "What nature?" some will say. "We might as well talk about the human relationship to nature in the context of cosmetics; isn't the point to get beyond the limits of nature?"

It is nonetheless the case, though, that the human relationship to nature is felt as especially important in the context of agriculture. If food were merely packages of nutrients, to be assessed solely on grounds of health and safety, the objections to GM foods would dissolve. As Mark Sagoff has written, "It is the classifications of social life—not those of biological science—that clothe food and everything else with meaning."[29] And among the social classifications are claims about the relationship with nature. Many people express through their food choices their relationship to nature. And they want this not just because how they eat is a convenient and effective way of signaling their relationship to nature. They want it, argues Michael Pollan, because

> the way we eat represents our most profound engagement with the natural world. Daily, our eating turns nature into culture, transforming the body of the world into our bodies and minds. Agriculture has done more to reshape the natural world than anything else we humans do, both its landscapes and the composition of its flora and fauna. Our eating also represents a relationship with dozens of other species—plants, animals, and fungi—with which we have evolved to the point where our fates are deeply entwined.... Eating puts us in touch with all that we share with the other animals, and all that sets us apart. It defines us.[30]

Thus, where food comes from and what has happened to it along the way, whether food *seems natural,* matters to people. At stake, then, in the decision to avoid GM foods (or, for that matter, in a decision actively to seek them) is a feeling about the kind of relationship to the natural world one wants to stand in.

So, how to make sense of it? Can the social classifications of food be defended? If the human relationship to nature in agriculture is not based on the ideal of *preservation*, then on what is it based? Sagoff's suggestion is that natural foods are those that possess a kind of "authenticity," as contrasted to being specious, illusory, or superficial. The natural is the unadorned—"trustworthy and honest...expressive of the virtues of rustic or peasant life." [31] Sagoff means to register an aesthetic point, not a moral claim. Part of what is appealing about the Humean account of morality, though, is that, if moral values are grounded in human sentiment, then it becomes possible to see moral values as blending into deeply motivating aesthetic reasons. Such aesthetic considerations can lie very close to one's views about what gives life point and depth. Food choices, including a decision to avoid GM foods, can be connected with a sense of cultural identity. Perhaps part of the reason Europeans have been more reluctant than Americans to accept GM foods is that the quality, variety, and preparation of food from particular sources in particular ways is sometimes intimately associated with European cultures.

The idea of natural as what is "authentic," "honest," or "unadorned" seems to rely subtly on some further point about nature—a point, I think, about the extent or form of human involvement in nature. To be authentic is to be the real thing, and to be honest is to represent something as it really is; to avoid adorning something is not to hang other things on it. In short, to be natural in this sense is not to have been altered *too much* or in the *wrong way*. Everything in the garden reveals and relies on human alteration. The question is how to do it honestly.

This is the question that has animated Pollan's proposal (discussed in Chapter 5) that the human relationship to nature be guided by a "gardener's ethic" rather than by a preservationist ethic. As Pollan sees it, nature "abhors a garden" yet nonetheless participates in it. A garden, suggests Pollan, works best when it draws from and learns from nature, when it channels nature toward human ends. In a garden, the ideal human relationship to nature is not preservation of nature, but a kind of exchange with nature. "Gardening was a subtle process of give and take with the landscape, a search for a middle ground between nature and culture."[32] A garden contrasts, for Pollan, both with a wilderness—nature as it once was but is no longer—and with a lawn—"nature under culture's boot...nature purged of sex and death."[33] A garden is "a place that admits of both nature and human habitation. But it is not, as I had imagined, a harmonious compromise between the two, nor is it stable;...it requires continuous human intervention or else it will collapse. The question for the gardener—and in a way it's a question for all of us—is, What is the proper character of that intervention?"[34] The exchange with nature comes across as a sort of conversation with nature, but a conversation that balances accepting, learning from, and even celebrating nature with a fair amount of arguing with nature, for the gardener has "a legitimate quarrel with nature—her weeds and storms and plagues, her rot and death."[35]

So, what about GM foods? Do they fit within the "proper character" of human interventions into nature, if we understand that character as a kind of respectful if sometimes combative conversation? "This is a vexed question," writes Thompson. Current biotechnology, he allows, certainly seems to be at odds with it: "the history of political conflict over agricultural research during the 1980s and 1990s shows that biotechnology and natural farming are like oil and water."[36] But as with the concept of "natural food," some of what is said about genetic engineering can be easily dismissed: in particular, if we give up the idea that the genes are the keys to an organism's essence— the defining characteristics of the kind which a given individual is meant to instantiate—then we will not regard genetic engineering as inherently evil.

Even setting such misconceptions aside, however, modifying an organism's genes is still arguably qualitatively different from other interventions. The usual point lodged against GM organisms is that the genetic rearrangements possible through gene transfer are much more radical than those possible through breeding. With breeding, one is stuck with manipulating a species' existing genetic pool, combining genes from closely related species, and waiting for chance mutations; with the technologies for GM, genes can be moved across kingdoms and phyla. Also, breeding involves a different kind of relationship with the organisms one is modifying. Breeders merely *select* from genotypes that are already given. The emergence of a new cultivar (a cultivated variety of a plant) through traditional breeding can be seen both from the human perspective and from what Pollan calls a "plant's eye perspective"; humans see breeding as creation of a natural resource, but the plants can "see" it as the creation of a new ecological niche, which the plants are "trying" (evolving) to exploit.[37] "The plant in its wildness proposes new qualities, and then man...selects which of those qualities will survive and prosper."[38] Thus does Pollan square breeding with the idea of a conversation with nature. In the development of a GM organism, however, the agronomist directly inserts the desired genetic variation. The causal story looks like a more one-sided relationship: human beings act on the organism, the organism is simply shaped. The Darwinian story of an organism evolving to fill a niche falls out of the picture.

The conversational ideal for the human relationship to nature is certainly a *social* classification. It seems to depend on social convention even more obviously than does the preservationist ideal, which I defended as a reasonable ideal to keep in mind in environmental affairs. The preservationist ideal rests on an understanding of nature that is social convention informed by empiricism; the conversational ideal seems less well grounded in empirical understanding of the world. What counts as a balanced exchange with nature? The concept strikes me as comprehensible and coherent, but it is very far from self-evident.

It is interesting to ask, for example, whether all kinds of genetic engineering are on par with each other if we compare them in light of the conversational ideal. Rollin notes that the concern about the naturalness of genetic engineering "seems to increase in direct proportion to the dramatic nature of the genetic intervention. If one is putting a human gene into an animal, or vice versa, or genetically creating 'monsters,' that is, creatures whose phenotype is markedly different from the parent stock, one is much likelier to occasion this response than if one is causing subtle genetic changes, for example, introducing the poll (hornlessness) gene into cattle."[39] The genetic change that has been introduced into salmon to cause them to grow faster is another example of a fairly minor tweaking; only a few genes are introduced into the salmon, and they are from fish (one of them from another salmon, in fact). Perhaps changes like this can be assimilated better to the conversational ideal. Once we have given up the idea that genetic interventions are on a completely different footing from other ways of manipulating an organism, it is open to us to have different views about different kinds of genetic changes.

Thompson's idea, in declaring that the question of the naturalness of GM foods is "vexed," is that the best way to understand "natural" in the context of farming is to see it as referring to a kind of craftsmanship, meaning something like "working with the natural properties of a thing, as when a carpenter planes wood 'with the grain.' To farm "naturally," in this sense, is to pay attention to the natural properties of one's plants, one's land, the weather, the insects and so on, and to use them to grow the crops and use the land in the best way possible—to alter nature "naturally." This sense of "naturally," which Thompson calls "artisanal," does not seem far removed from Pollan's notion of the conversational relationship to nature that a gardener strives to maintain: both notions have one working *with* nature. But Thompson goes on to argue that there is a sense in which genetic technologies *could* be "natural," even if current biotechnology does not seem that way: "one can view the detailed mapping of plant genomes as enhancing our collective capacity to farm 'with the grain,' since genomics allows a better understanding of the fine grain of genetic capabilities in agricultural plants.... [thus permitting] farming approaches that are far more sensitive to the array of situational characteristics and variables important in artisanal farming."[40]

There's another way in which the generality of the objection to genetic engineering might be limited, given a conversational rather than an essentialist understanding of that objection. Suppose genetic technology could

help us create blight-resistant American chestnuts that were phenotypi-
cally indistinguishable from "natural" American chestnuts, with the excep-
tion that they survive whereas "natural" American chestnuts are mostly
dead and dying. Eastern forests that have only "natural" trees are forests
with an "unnatural" mix of species. Maybe, on balance, even those who are
troubled by human genetic alteration of other species would find this an
acceptable exercise of it. I would. In short, there might be cases in which
GM organisms can be used to *restore* nature; concerns about their naturalness might be offset by benefits to nature.

I argued in Chapter 5 that the gardener's ethic is less illuminating for
the human relationship to nature than a preservationist ethic and that it
is not the ethic I would like to employ to guide environmental protection.
A gardener works with nature but not necessarily on nature's behalf. But is
the ethic right for *agriculture*? It probably does not provide very much more
pointed guidance in this domain than in the environmental. The ideal of a
"conversation" with nature is straightforwardly metaphorical, and which
human interventions into nature fit with it and which sit poorly with it
is vague. Perhaps genetic engineering sits less well with it than does, say,
the propagation of heirloom cultivars. In another place, Pollan describes
his experimentation with growing NewLeaf potatoes and his ambivalence
about them. He found he could not condemn them, but he also never
brought himself to eat them. They sat in perpetual storage in his house.
In my own life, I pay very little attention to whether the foods I buy in the
store include GM organisms, but my garden counts as "organic" (for most
crops, most years), and my plantings emphasize heirloom varieties.

What the gardening ethic tells against more clearly is probably the overall
industrial agricultural mindset within which GM foods have found a niche.
I have always assumed that when Prince Charles lamented that GM technologies raised a question of whether we would condone the "industrialisation
of Life," his point was that genetic modification *is* a kind of industrialization
of life, but maybe the point was really that it would lead that way. Maybe
the better stance would be to object to GM only insofar as it contributes
to industrialization. What is objectionable about industrial agriculture
from the perspective of someone who cares about the human relationship
to nature is not the fact of doing agriculture on a big scale, but the way
it is usually done *when* done on a big scale. In the industrial agricultural
mindset, crops are grown as vast monocultures quite unlike anything that
would be found in nature, and they are highly vulnerable to diseases, pests,
and fluctuations in the weather. An organic agricultural mindset encourages the farmer to plant a variety of crops and varieties, both discouraging
vast outbreaks of diseases and pests and limiting the farmer's exposure to

any one crop failure. ("Organic" agriculture can itself shift toward an industrial mindset, however, even while adhering to the USDA restrictions on "organic" farming.[41]) The industrial agricultural mindset also encourages the use of applied fertilizers over measures to improve the soil itself. (After visiting an organic potato farm, Pollan describes the soil as completely different from the "uniform grayish powder" he had seen at other farms in the area. "The difference, I understood, was that this soil was alive. Much more than an inert mechanism for conducting water and chemicals to the crops, it actually contributed nutrients of its own making to the plants."[42]) In short, the industrial paradigm endorses a manufacturing over an ecological paradigm. Although featuring technological sophistication, it is really fundamentally about simplicity, about trying to iron out the irregularities of nature and ignoring the complexities that careful organic farming is based on.[43] It is about control of nature, with practices that fly in the face of natural mechanisms and must be strenuously maintained over against nature, rather than about collaboration with nature. It is also, it could be added, about automation rather than labor and corporate instead of family and community structure.

With animals, too, industrial agriculture tends to depart from nature, at least in the sense that it encourages farmers to treat their animals in ways that have ever less to do with animal husbandry, with caring for animals, and more to do with productivity. Animals are squeezed together into tight spaces, denied opportunities to engage in species-typical behavior, fed what makes them grow fastest and most economically rather than what they want to eat or what's good for them, and goosed with hormones that make them more productive. And, of course, in an industrial mindset, there is no thought of retiring an old and unproductive milk cow to the end of the barn; that would be a relic of the Yorkshire farms in *All Creatures Great and Small*. In an industrial mindset, inefficient animals must be killed. The moral problem with such treatment can be couched most forcefully in terms of the harm done to animals, of course, and, indeed, one way of dealing with the harm might be to engineer them genetically so that they accept living in industrial conditions or at least are incapable of suffering from them.[44] I suspect this will strike many as an unfortunate way of solving the problem, though—a capitulation to the industrialization of Life.

FOOD POLICY

The moral case offered, then, is that the ideal human relationship to nature, in agriculture, is best understood not as *preservation* of nature but as a kind of balance in the alteration of nature—a "conversation" with nature. What makes a food "natural" (or "organic") is not that humans did not produce it, but that its production reflects a kind of limited exchange with nature, one in which nature is not thoroughly dominated. The stance is allegiance to a metaphor, to be sure, but a metaphor that might well matter greatly. Pollan, once again: "The metaphors we use to describe the natural world strongly influence the way we approach it, the style and extent of our attempts at control. It makes all the difference in (and to) the world if one conceives of a farm as a factory or a forest as a farm. Now [with GM foods] we're about to find out what happens when people begin approaching the genes of our food plants as software."[45]

A person who is committed to living in conversation with nature can plausibly think of consuming GM foods as sitting uncomfortably with that commitment, given how the evolutionary story—the "plant's eye" perspective—gives way to a story centering on human control. But we can scarcely say that someone who disagrees with that view is obtuse. The case is just not that strong. What we have is not a general case against GM foods so much as simply a defense of a personal stand against GM foods: it is a reasonable way of expressing an ideal by which one might well want to live. It is Pollan growing GM potatoes, deciding they're not reprehensible, but not finding them choiceworthy.

The next step, of course, is to figure out how public life accommodates that private ideal. Since we do not all produce our own food but rely on large social systems to produce and distribute it, the ideal cannot be honored alone. There are two issues, I think. First is figuring out how to reach some sort of consensus on what the ideal calls for—how to deal with the ineradicable fuzziness of it. The second issue is, in a way, figuring out how to go forward without consensus—how to let those who hold the ideal do so without imposing it on those who do not.

Lines and Lists

If we have given up on talking about preserving *pure* nature, then the concern that the distinction is impossible gives way to a concern about precisely where and how to draw the line between "natural" and "unnatural." Many meals could exemplify "unnatural" for us. My favorite example is Tang—the "orange-flavored drink" that became popular after American astronauts took it to space with them. As I write this chapter, the fast-food chain Taco Bell has been charged with using a "meat filling" instead of meat in its tacos and burritos, while nonetheless merely calling it "meat." The "meat filling" reportedly has various "extenders" to help it take up space. The base case is presumably something like the dinner that Pollan once called "the Perfect Meal"—"perfect" not because it was good (although he thought it was) but because "this labor- and thought-intensive dinner, enjoyed in the company of fellow foragers, gave me the opportunity, so rare in modern life, to eat in full consciousness of everything involved in feeding myself."[46] The Perfect Meal was the meal with the shortest possible route to the dinner table, and one in which every step of production was known in detail and could be borne in mind while eating. Food was either collected from the wild (Pollan gives the reader many pages about foraging for mushrooms), hunted (Pollan shot a boar), or grown. Food that is merely gathered seems the very purest case: in principle, one might sometimes just lower one's head and chew the food right off the ground, so that the human intervention is nothing more than mastication and digestion. How far away from the purest case—how much and what kinds of human production are still consistent with the label "natural," and in particular what we should say about genetic interventions—is what we need to articulate. Pollan's Perfect Meal includes food grown in the garden, but gardens, of course, are abhorred by nature.

First, we should say something about what the case will look like—how we will go about drawing the line. Very likely, the defense will often be inadequate: if we agree that, in between reasonably clear cases at either end of the spectrum, there is a gray area, then there is no perfect criterion for sorting out the cases in the gray area. Those cases just are variously underdetermined or indeterminate. Nonetheless, some sort of line drawing will be necessary; eventually, the shopper must push the cart down the grocery aisle and decide what's for dinner, and if the human relationship to nature is important, then the shopper must decide, item by item, what to put in the cart. Moreover, these decisions will effectively associate everything in the gray area with one end or the other of the spectrum. About everything that seems indeterminate, the shopper must say either, "It might be okay, but I think I'll skip it," or "I suppose this can pass": if no decision can be made about a particular jar of pickles, then either the shopper concludes that the value of the human relationship to nature is suspended, or he decides to play it safe and steer clear of the indeterminate cases. In short, the line drawing will be somewhat arbitrary.

If there is no single clear rule for marking what falls inside and outside the use of the concept, and if the final line drawing is somewhat arbitrary, then a list of the decisions one makes will be, to some degree, just that—a list. And, in fact, this is exactly what happens. In the United States, the primary authority on what counts as "natural" in agriculture

is the USDA, through its "organic" certification. The FDA generally dis-
courages use of the term "natural," on grounds that almost any food has
been processed and even minimal processing is contrary to "natural," but
it nonetheless allows food to be called "natural" if the food contains no
added color, artificial flavors, or synthetic substances. It has no policy
on "organic." The USDA also has a relatively modest policy on "natural": meat and poultry products may be called natural, for example, when
they contain no artificial or synthetic ingredients and are only minimally
processed. On the topic of "organic" agriculture, however, the USDA has
much to say. USDA regulations set out a "National List of Allowed and
Prohibited Substances" to stipulate what is compatible with the term.[47]
By and large, "organic" produce must be produced and handled without
the use of synthetic substances, but some synthetic substances have
been deemed acceptable. To control insects, for example, it is acceptable
to use fixed coppers, such as copper hydroxide, if the use of the material
minimizes accumulation in the soil. Also acceptable are hydrated lime,
hydrogen peroxide, and potassium bicarbonate. Streptomycin may be
used to control fire blight in apples and pears, but that is, at this writing,
its only acceptable use.

A list-making strategy is useless, of course, unless a critical mass can
agree on a list. Perhaps this is why lists are produced by groups. Since
reason alone cannot compel agreement, reason is augmented by social
authority: people come together through government agencies such as
the USDA, or private associations such as Certified Naturally Grown, not
merely to defend a moral line, but to decide where the line should be.[48] Of
course, social authority alone cannot produce fully dispositive judgments
about how words are appropriately used or what moral judgments are correct. However, the list-making body can acquire authority by convention
within a delimited domain: those within the domain can simply grant the
list-making body authority to make certain decisions about what will count
as natural, or the list-making body may acquire it through democratic
processes.

In effect, these lists are attempts to work through a range of examples
and, in so doing, to stipulate more precise understandings of what is inherently vague. The generation of these lists is not cut loose from the guidance of reason—it can be guided both by some general principles and by
analogical reasoning from case to case—but the arbitrariness of the lone
shopper is not eliminated either. Another group of decision makers might
well come up with another list.

The same strategy is followed, incidentally, to sort natural from unnatural
ways of improving human bodies in sports—of delimiting acceptable diet

and training regimens from doping and other enhancement techniques. The World Anti-Doping Agency (WADA), for example, regularly updates a "Prohibited List" of substances that athletes may not use if they want to compete in sports events that are governed by groups that adhere to WADA standards; the International Association of Athletics Federations, which governs most track and field events, is one such.[49]

Labels

Plainly, not only would some people write the list differently, but others simply will not attach much significance to any list. Some people may not connect the human relationship to nature with what gives their life meaning, or they may value a very different relationship to nature—one that celebrates human understanding and ingenuity and leaves them unconcerned about GM food. In principle, a person might even take a special delight in that use of human capacities. There are competing ideals at play, as I suggested in Chapter 3.

Some may also favor Pollan's "conversational" relationship to nature yet attach limited significance to genetic modification. The genes are not special repositories of moral value, and some applications of the technology might seem worth tolerating after all. A person who wishes to avoid GM foods herself might still sensibly decide to promote a GM food that could stave off famine in Africa. Many mice used in medical research are genetically engineered to have certain traits, but the fact that, according to the considerations given earlier, they are not natural may seem beside the point.

All of this suggests that the policy response to GM food should be a compromise: the policy should make it possible for people to uphold their commitments but should not force others to conform to them. We should carve out room for rejection of GM foods yet not reject them universally. In the Rawlsian language of the GM food policy that Robert Streiffer and Thomas Hedemann have elucidated, the objection to GM foods falls outside society's "overlapping consensus" of reasonable moral and philosophical worldviews,[50] and aggressively oppositional policies such as outright bans cannot be justified (assuming, of course, that the foods are safe). At the same time, though, food policy proposals that would force citizens to relinquish their commitment to natural foods also cannot be justified.

The way to strike this compromise is probably through some form of labeling. Labeling food as made from or including GM organisms would allow people to avoid, ignore, or deliberately select those foods, thereby living by their values without imposing them on others. The long-standing policy of the FDA, however, is that food labels are only for informing consumers about substances in a product that may affect consumers' health and safety; since there is no evidence that GM foods present a safety concern, "the agency does not believe that the method of development of a new plant variety...is normally material information" that should be disclosed on a label.[51] There is, in fact, some reason to ask about the nutritional quality and safety of GM foods since, given the complexity of organisms, a gene can have slightly different effects in different organisms.[52] But there is greater reason to wonder about the FDA's claim that labels should touch only on safety issues. In fact, that does not seem to be true. Labels frequently tell consumers something about *where food comes from*, even when there are no safety or health considerations at stake. Orange juice that is produced from concentrate rather than from "fresh-squeezed" oranges must be labeled as "produced from concentrate," for example.[53] Also, the Food, Drug, and Cosmetic Act requires that labels indicate "the name and place of business of the manufacturer, packer, or distributor."[54] A food's provenance is not a property of the food itself; it is what Robert Streiffer and Alan Rubel have called a "relational property" between food and those who consume it.[55] The fact that a food is "natural" is also, in part, a question about provenance, and it is also, in part, an important relational property between consumers and food: it allows consumers to carry out, through their eating, the relationship they wish to have with nature.

This exchange does not end the discussion about labeling. Some questions remain unresolved:[56] Should the labeling of GM foods be voluntary or mandatory? What should the labels identify—food that lacks GM ingredients or food that contains them? Can they let producers trumpet a selling point, or should they convey information discreetly? Moreover, labeling might prove to be so onerous and expensive for producers as to outweigh the good of protecting consumers' ability to act on their commitments— although the good in question seems significant and industry's misgivings about new product regulations regularly turn out to be inflated. Nor would a discussion about food labels be the end of the matter on GM food policy. It is also necessary, for example, to figure out how organic and conventional farms can coexist. Conventional farms that grow GM foods sometimes produce pollen that contains the genetic change and can drift into neighboring farms; if that happens, the neighbor's produce may not count as "organic." Somehow or other, though, coexistence seems possible, and it is all that a stand against GM foods warrants.

NOTES

1. Paul B. Thompson, *Food Biotechnology in Ethical Perspective* (London, U.K.: Blackie Academic & Professional, 1997), 211.
2. Andrew Kimbrell and Jeremy Rifkin, "Biotechnology—A Proposal for Regulatory Reform," *Notre Dame Journal of Law, Ethics, and Public Policy* 3 (1987), 117–43, at 126, quoted in Thompson, *Food Biotechnology in Ethical Perspective*, 211.
3. Edie Lau, "'Glofish' Won't Be Lighting Up the State," *The Sacramento Bee*, December 4, 2003.
4. Charles, Prince of Wales, "Questions About Genetically Modified Organisms," *Daily Mail*, June 1, 1999.
5. Bernice Bovenkerk, Frans W. A. Brom, and Babs J. van den Bergh, "Brave New Birds: The Use of 'Animal Integrity' in Animal Ethics," *Hastings Center Report* 32, no. 1 (2002), 16–22, at 16.
6. William Hallman, Wilfred Hebden, Cara Cuite, Helen Aquino, and John Lang, "Americans and GM Food: Knowledge, Opinion, and Interest in 2004," New Brunswick, N.J.: Food Policy Institute, Cook College, Rutgers—The State University of New Jersey, 2004; available at http://www.foodpolicyinstitute. org/docs/reports/NationalStudy2004.pdf.
7. Pew Initiative on Food and Biotechnology, "Public Sentiment About Genetically Modified Food," Pew Initiative on Food and Biotechnology, 2005; available at http://pewagbiotech.org/research/2005update/1.php.
8. Jennifer Sosin and Mark David Richards, "What Will Consumers Do? Understanding Consumer Response when Meat and Milk from Cloned Animals Reach Supermarkets," Washington, D.C.: KRC Research, 2005; available at http://www.krcresearch.com/selectReports.html.
9. International Food Information Council, "IFIC survey: Food Biotechnology not a Top-of-Mind Concern for American Consumers," 2005; available at http://www. ific.org/research/upload/2005BiotechSurvey.pdf.
10. Claire Marris, Brian Wynne, Peter Simmons, and Sue Weldon, "Public Perceptions of Agricultural Biotechnologies in Europe: Final report of the PABE Research Project," funded by the Commission of European Communities, 2001. Emphasis in original.
11. Thompson, Food Biotechnology in Ethical Perspective, 215.
12. Bernard E. Rollin, *The Frankenstein Syndrome: Ethical and Social Issues in the Genetic Engineering of Animals* (New York, Cambridge: Cambridge University Press, 1995), 21.
13. Rollin, *The Frankenstein Syndrome*, 66.
14. Michael Pollan, *Second Nature: A Gardener's Education* (New York: Grove Press, 1991), 37.
15. United States Department of Agriculture, Economic Research Service, "Adoption of Genetically Engineered Crops in the U.S.," http://www.ers.usda.gov/Data/ BiotechCrops/, accessed February 12, 2011.
16. Erik Stokstand, "USDA Decides Against New Regulation of GM Crops," *Science* 331 (February 4, 2011), 523.
17. Food and Drug Administration, "Completed Consultations on Bioengineered Foods," available at http://www.fda.gov/default.htm; Pew Initiative on Food and Biotechnology, "Application of Biotechnology for Functional Foods," Pew Initiative on Food and Biotechnology, 2007; available at http://www.pewtrusts.

org/uploadedFiles/wwwpewtrustsorg/Reports/Food_and_Biotechnology/ PIFB_Functional_Foods.pdf.

18. Committee on the Impact of Biotechnology Farm-Level Economics and Sustainability, National Research Council, The Impact of Genetically Engineered Crops on Farm Sustainability in the United States (Washington, D.C.: National Academy of Sciences, 2010), 3.

19. Craig Holdrege and Steve Talbott, *Beyond Biotechnology: The Barren Promise of Genetic Engineering* (Lexington: University Press of Kentucky, 2008), 9.

20. Andrew Pollack, "Genetically Altered Salmon Gets Closer to the Table," *New York Times*, June 25, 2010.

21. "Glofish: Experience the Glow!" http://www.glofish.com/.

22. Holdrege and Talbott, *Beyond Biotechnology*, 33.

23. Denis Noble, *The Music of Life: Biology Beyond the Genome* (Oxford, U.K.: Oxford University Press, 2006).

24. Holmes Rolston III, "What Do We Mean by the Intrinsic Value and Integrity of Plants and Animals?" in *Genetic Engineering and the Intrinsic Value and Integrity of Animals and Plants*, proceedings of a workshop at the Royal Botanic Garden, ed. David Heaf and Johannes Wirz (Switzerland: International Forum for Genetic Engineering, 2002), 5–10, at 6.

25. Rolston, "What Do We Mean?" 6

26. Ibid., 5.

27. Ibid., 6.

28. Rollin, *The Frankenstein Syndrome*, 36.

29. Mark Sagoff, "Genetic Engineering and the Concept of the Natural," in *Genetic Prospects: Essays on Biotechnology, Ethics, and Public Policy*, ed. V.V. Gearing (Oxford, U.K.: Rowman & Littlefield, 2003), 27–25, 24.

30. Pollan, *The Omnivore's Dilemma*, 10.

31. Sagoff, "Genetic Engineering and the Concept of the Natural," 18.

32. Pollan, *Second Nature*, 62.

33. Ibid.

34. Ibid., 49.

35. Ibid., 193.

36. Paul Thompson, "Unnatural Farming and the Debate over Genetic Manipulation," in *Genetic Prospects: Essays on Biotechnology, Ethics, and Public Policy*, ed. V.V. Gearing (Oxford, U.K.: Rowman & Littlefield, 2003), 27–40, at 32.

37. Michael Pollan, *The Botany of Desire: A Plant's Eye View of the World* (New York: Random House, 2001).

38. Ibid., 196.

39. Rollin, *The Frankenstein Syndrome*, 21.

40. Thompson, "Unnatural Farming," 33–34.

41. Michael Pollan, *The Omnivore's Dilemma: A Natural History of Four Meals* (New York: Penguin Books, 2006), 134ff.

42. Pollan, *Botany of Desire*, 223.

43. Holdrege and Talbott, *Beyond Biotechnology*, 10.

44. Rollin, *The Frankenstein Syndrome*, 169ff.

45. Pollan, *Botany of Desire*, 191.

46. Michael Pollan, *The Omnivore's Dilemma*, 9.

47. United States Department of Agriculture, Agricultural Marketing Service, "National List of Allowed and Prohibited Substances," available at http://www. ams.usda.gov; accessed February 5, 2010.

48. Certified Naturally Grown, home page, http://www.naturallygrown.org/.
49. World Anti-Doping Agency, "The World Anti-Doping Code; The 2013 Prohibited List," Available at http://www.wada-ama.org/Documents/World_ Anti-Doping_Program/WADP-Prohibited-list/2013/WADA-Prohibited-List-2013-EN.pdf.
50. Robert Streiffer and T. Hedemann, "The Political Import of Intrinsic Objections to Genetically Engineered Food," *Journal of Agriculture and Environmental Ethics* 18 (2004), 191–210.
51. United States Department of Health and Human Services, Food and Drug Administration, "Statement of Policy—Foods Derived from New Plant Varieties," Federal Register 57, no. 104 (1992), 22984; available at http://www.fda.gov/ Food/GuidanceRegulation/GuidanceDocumentsRegulatoryInformation/ Biotechnology/ucm096095.htm.
52. Holdrege and Talbott, *Beyond Biotechnology*, 42–56.
53. Ibid., 44–45.
54. FDCA sec. 343(e).
55. Robert Streiffer and Alan Rubel, "Democratic Principles and Mandatory Labeling of Genetically Engineered Food," *Public Affairs Quarterly* 18, no. 3 (2004), 223–48.
56. United States Department of Health and Human Services, Food and Drug Administration, Center for Food Safety and Applied Nutrition, "Voluntary Labeling Indicating Whether Foods Have or Have Not Been Developed Using Bioengineering," draft guidance, 2001; available at: http://www.fda.gov/ Food/GuidanceComplianceRegulatoryInformation/GuidanceDocuments/ FoodLabelingNutrition/UCM059098.

CHAPTER 7

Nature in the Factory

Synthetic Biology

With some scientific and technological developments, the public gets excited when the technology hits the streets and generates new products and services. Radio caught the public's attention when radios became available. The Internet had been in the works for some years before most people even knew about it. But with developments in biology, the excitement tends to precede the application. In the 1990s, genetic engineering was going to cure the incurable; 15 years on, there are only a few scattered reports of success, and these only on a few individuals at a time and not completely smoothly (the treatment sometimes led to cancer). In 2000, when the Human Genome Project succeeded in completing the first draft of the human genome, the results were going to change medicine; 10 years later, the *New York Times* ran a story about how meager the results were.[1] With embryonic stem cells, we are now just past the first flush of excitement, and there's no reason to be disappointed that new cell-based treatments have not gone into clinical use yet. Still, it's plain that excitement preceded success by many years—assuming that there *is* success somewhere down the road.

Anyone who has observed this history can be forgiven for adopting a wait-and-see attitude toward "synthetic biology," which, in the past few years, has been identified as the next big "revolution" in biology. With synthetic biology, we are still in the first flush. However, there are reasons to think that some lines of work in synthetic biology might come to fruition and could have a far-reaching impact. To date anyway, synthetic biology focuses on simpler organisms. And because the organisms are so simple, there are no concerns about obtaining their informed consent to the research nor even about harming them, and therefore some of the regulatory hurdles that impede research on stem cell therapies don't apply to synthetic biology. The prospect that the technology might actually be successful raises other ethical questions, however, including questions about how synthetic biology might change the human relationship to nature.

A fully adequate way of articulating this concern has been as elusive in the context of synthetic biology as anywhere else. Some speak of whether it is appropriate for humans to take on the task of "creating life" and whether, by doing so, they aren't "playing god," which has led to some heavy sighing and eye-rolling among the proponents of synthetic biology. One leading figure in the field has asserted that "the questions of playing God or not are so superficial and embarrassingly simple that they're not going to be useful."[2] In the introduction to *What Is Life?*, which tracks a particularly provocative line of research in synthetic biology, Ed Regis, a science writer and philosopher by training, agrees that the field raises moral, political, and legal questions, but mocks most of what has been said about them: "The problems started with the perennial and trite layman's taunt, the claim that creating life was 'playing God.'"[3]

I will argue here for a middle way on the "playing god" concern about synthetic biology. We should take it seriously. This will mean exploring and examining the concern—trying to articulate it more clearly. I will argue that, at least with respect to synthetic biology, claims about "playing god" turn out to stand for several different but related objections that need to be considered individually. They are all interesting and potentially sophisticated positions. Some of them, but not all, lend themselves well to the development of public policy. For synthetic biology, however, none of them really makes a difference for public policy—at least, not for synthetic biology as it stands now. If the field turns out to be as powerful as some envision, perhaps matters will change.

FROM UNDERSTANDING TO ENGINEERING

The barrage of scholarly reports and media coverage about how synthetic biology will change the world gives the impression that it is a specific and recent milestone. "Synthetic biology is another transformative innovation" in biology, begin Jonathan Tucker and Raymond Zilinskas, comparable in significance to the discovery of the structure of DNA, the deciphering of the genetic code, and the development of genetic engineering (recombinant

DNA) technology.[4] Exactly what synthetic biology *is*, however, is itself debated.

Many commentators describe synthetic biology very broadly as a new way of *doing* biology: synthetic biology is the attempt to engineer biological constructs—parts, systems, organisms—to serve particular human functions. A banner across the top of a community web site (started by people at Harvard University and the Massachusetts Institute of Technology and maintained collectively by people in synthetic biology) declares that synthetic biology is just "(a) the design and construction of new biological parts, devices, and systems, and (b) the re-design of existing, natural biological systems for useful purposes." But using an understanding of biology to construct things is not new at all, leading some scientists to wonder what the label "synthetic biology" really means.[5] Arguably, it is just a new label for essentially the same technology used to create genetically modified crops and animals in agriculture. Even within the field that calls itself synthetic biology, it is a commonplace that synthetic work can be traced to 1828, when the German chemist Friedrich Wöhler figured out a way to make synthetic urea. If one emphasizes the continuity of synthetic biology with older forms of genetic engineering, what's new is merely that our understanding of biology has progressed to the point that, combined with ever faster and more powerful tools for manipulating biological systems— in particular, machines to synthesize medium-length strings of DNA—the possibilities for construction are vastly greater.

Engineering is certainly the core idea behind the label. Traditional biology has been "analytic"; it has been about understanding life as it is. "Synthetic" biology is aimed at constructing what might be. Drew Endy, a synthetic biologist at Stanford University and a leading figure in the field, has noted, "if you consider nature to be a machine, you can see that it is not perfect and that it can be revised and improved."[6] A report from the Rathenau Instituut, a Dutch organization that specializes in technology assessment, describes the difference in revolutionary language: "Until recently, biotechnologists focused on modifying the DNA of existing organisms (genetic modification). Synthetic biologists go one step further. They want to design new life and construct this from scratch."[7]

In principle, defining synthetic biology merely in terms of building recognizes no limits to the kinds of biological systems or organisms we might work on. Complex, multicellular organisms engineered to do what we want can be envisioned: gourds that grow big enough to be used as dwellings or rats that sniff out and attack unexploded ordinance. In practice, however, synthetic biology is about the creation or modification of individual cells, and it is chiefly about the creation or modification of single-celled organisms—that level of life that scientists stand the best chance of being able to "engineer" and which industrialists stand the best chance of being able to use. What microbes do with their lives is basically a matter of biochemistry: take these chemical and energy inputs and produce those outputs. An engineered microbe can therefore be a kind of biological factory.

In one way, then, synthetic biology is agricultural biotechnology taken down to its rudiments, down to the simplest possible organisms. In another way, it is ag biotech taken to higher levels. Work in it can be described as advancing along four broad lines (although taxonomies for the field are debated nearly as much as definitions): biobricks development, genome synthesis, research on novel biologies, and advanced genetic modification. I give "biobricks development"—or what some commentators have called "DNA-based device construction"[8]—pride of place as the first line because it arguably best exemplifies an engineering mindset. Biobricks are standardized, interchangeable genetic sequences that, if inserted into a cell's genes, should reliably cause the cell to function in specific, well-characterized ways. A microbe could be modified to sense the presence of a chemical, trigger a metabolic pathway, and then generate a certain output, for example, simply by pulling together a set of biobricks—off-the-shelf genetic parts, as it were—that "code" for these various steps. Synthetic biology could then be carried out much faster and by many more people; it would depend less on esoteric insight into how genes work than on access to the catalogs in which the needed genetic parts are explained and sold.

A second line, synthetic genomics, works toward the engineering of organisms from the end opposite the biobricks model. It aims at the simplification and fabrication of whole genomes, rather than parts. The goal is to design and build a "minimal genome," one containing the minimum amount of genetic material needed to sustain life and capable of serving as a kind of chassis or platform that could be augmented with more specialized genetic sequences to create organisms with desirable properties. In principle, synthetic genomics and biobricks development are complementary approaches: one could augment a minimal genome with bioparts. Synthetic genomics is associated most closely with the J. Craig Venter Institute (JCVI), which has reported several milestones in synthesizing cells with a minimal genome, all involving species of the bacterial genus *Mycoplasma*, whose members already have extremely small and presumably nearly minimal genomes.[9] In 2006, scientists at JCVI reported that they had managed to identify which of the genes of the *M. genitalium* genome are "essential genes" and which are dispensable. In 2007, JCVI scientists reported that they extracted the genome from a *M. mycoides* cell and transplanted it into a *M. capricolum* cell whose genome had been removed. A 2008 article reported that the entire genome of *M. genitalium* had been synthesized. And, in 2010, JCVI announced it had combined the previous two developments: it had synthesized an entire *M. mycoides* genome and inserted it into a genome-less *M. capricolum* cell, ending up with a fully functioning *M. mycoides*. Collectively, the work is proof of principle that the fabrication of a living cell with a minimal genome should be possible.

Research on novel biology, a third broad line of work in synthetic biology, itself takes several disparate forms. Protocell development is like synthetic genomics in that it, too, aims at producing a simplified cellular platform or "chassis," but instead of starting with existing cellular genomes it tries to reconceive the overall set of biological structures and mechanisms necessary for cells—cell walls, intracellular transport, metabolism, and replication.[10] In principle, protocell development might use cellular materials and mechanisms different from those found in any existing organisms. For Regis, this is the ultimate goal: the creation of "a new form of life," "a genuinely new living entity, . . . one not based on biology and not made out of the customary biological ingredients: no DNA, no conventional biomolecules, no cell membrane of the ordinary type, no nucleus, no mitochondria, no endoplasmic reticulum or any of the other innumerable vital trappings of normal, orthodox biological cells."[11]

Protocell development is a form of synthetic biology that does not rely mainly on genetic science, but some other kinds of novel biologies are mind-bending forms of genetic science. Some molecular geneticists have proposed, for example, that novel genetic arrangements could be developed to augment or replace the existing lot: these might include nucleotides that do not exist in nature, codons (sets of three nucleotides) that are reassigned to create new kinds of amino acids, and nucleotides whose arrangement of atoms is the mirror image of what's found in existing nucleotides (so that DNA molecules would spiral in the opposite direction from what we see in nature).[12] The result would be DNA that behaved entirely differently from existing DNA; organisms with the new DNA might have different properties and produce new kinds of chemicals. The new kinds of DNA could be combined with existing DNA to create still more complicated biological systems, but they might also begin to inhabit a parallel biological universe. If an organism with mirror DNA turned out to be functional, for example, it could not reproduce sexually with any "natural" organism, nor could it be infected by existing viruses.

Finally, there are a number of disparate examples of research that are sometimes described as synthetic biology but that look more like extensions of what we might now think of as "traditional" genetic engineering, which is the technology behind GM crops and livestock. They consist in the modification of existing organisms with genes drawn from other sources, and, since they do not fit neatly into any of the categories just described, might as well just be called "advanced genetic modification." One example of this line of work is the modification of *Escherichia coli* and later (as the research progressed) baker's yeast to produce artemisinic acid, from which the antimalarial drug artemisinin can then be produced. The modification involves multiple genes from various organisms and the creation of a metabolic pathway that does not exist in nature—what is accomplished is arguably not just "transfer" but compilation or construction. The technology was further developed by Amyris Biotechnologies and then transferred to the pharmaceutical company Sanofi-Aventis.

Another example is the work being done on many different kinds of organisms to develop new ways of producing biofuel. As of the end of 2010, there were somewhere around a dozen firms and a major research endeavor funded by the US Department of Energy and led by the Lawrence Berkeley National Laboratory working on various strategies in various organisms—from bacteria that would turn complex sugars into biofuels to algae and cyanobacteria that would produce fuel using sunlight, carbon dioxide, and water. Both the production of artemisinic acid and the work on biofuels are emblematic of the combination of industrial and social benefit that many in synthetic biology hope for. At technical conferences in synthetic biology, it is held as a sort of truism too obvious to dwell on that the future of civilization may depend on the field's success. Perhaps the most significant of the social benefits is a partial solution to environmental problems, achieved both by replacing or supplementing more environmentally destructive industrial processes with more benign ones and by making possible new means of environmental remediation. Enthusiasts speak of organisms engineered to absorb carbon, clean up oil spills or toxic waste sites, or rebuild ocean food chains.

In short, synthetic biology is composed of disparate lines of work, usually but not necessarily involving DNA, united by the goal of redeploying biological science to foster biological engineering. It might someday lead to new kinds of organisms—protocell work could even produce a non–carbon-based, which is to say "nonorganic," biochemistry—but, for the time being, the work closest to producing actual applications is the fourth line, centering on making modifications to existing organisms. (For this kind of work especially, the label "synthetic biology" is a bit overblown, insofar as that term suggests that scientists are creating new kinds of life forms.) It might eventually be applicable to complex organisms, but, for the time being, it centers on the modification of single-cell organisms, with the caveat that modifying the single-cell organisms of the microbiome—the vast assemblages of single-cell organisms that live on, in, and with multicellular organisms—could be an indirect way of modifying the larger organism. (In mid-2013, work to insert some firefly genetic sequences into a mustard plant, creating a glowing plant, was being hailed—and lamented—as a significant new application of synthetic biology, although the work appears to be technically simple enough that it does not even count as "advanced" genetic engineering.) It is motivated partly by scientific curiosity and beneficial social goals, but driven economically by its promise of a wide array of industrial opportunities.

A NEW INDUSTRIAL AGE AND A SECOND CREATION

There is a growing consensus that the capacity synthetic biology gives us to modify and create organisms raises an assortment of ethical questions—none of them entirely new, but perhaps now arising in especially sharp forms. At the top of the list are the possible tangible consequences of synthetic biology for human lives. The potential benefit genuinely seems quite great: the work might provide scientific insight, new kinds of medicines and other products, and environmentally friendlier ways of producing many familiar products. At the same time, synthetic biology presents grave potential harms. Perhaps the most arresting of these are the possible malevolent uses of the technology: in theory, a rogue state or a well-funded bioterrorist could recreate smallpox or the influenza strain of the 1918–19 flu pandemic, or perhaps even create new kinds of pathogens, such as amped-up smallpox or a strain of H5N1 (also called bird flu) that could be transmitted from person to person. Another, more prosaic set of concerns centers on accidents—or what some have called "bioerrorism": synthesized organisms might escape from the laboratory or factory, turn out to have properties different from what was intended and predicted, perhaps mutate to acquire them, and become established in the wild, posing a threat to public health, agriculture, or the environment.[13] Finally, synthetic biology might turn out to have undesirable economic consequences. Synthetic biologists believe that the field is the beginning of a new industrial age in which cellular factories will obsolete many existing ways of producing and transporting goods. The critics worry that instead of correcting the problems of the industrial age, as proponents envision, those problems will only be worsened: cellular factories will destroy the livelihoods of people who now harvest or grow the products that the factories will someday manufacture, they will run on complex sugars extracted from sugarcane or other plants that displace food crops and damage the environment in vast tracts of the developing world, and they will concentrate the means of production in the hands of a very small set of capitalists who have managed to lay claim to the right patents.[14]

Intermixed with these concerns about the consequences of this new industrial age are concerns about the very idea of it—concerns, that is, about using living things as factories, about claiming living things as intellectual property, and generally about applying the principles of engineering to living things. Synthetic biology thus raises concerns about the human relationship to nature in a particularly interesting and sharp form. The concerns are not always objections. For synthetic biologists themselves, the work appears intrinsically good—a noble activity, in and of itself. The pursuit of science is the advancement of human mastery, and synthetic biology exemplifies human mastery especially dramatically: as Regis provocatively puts it, the creation of a brand new form of life amounts to a "second creation" that is brought about by human beings, to their everlasting credit. It is humanism in its grandest, maybe most self-aggrandizing form. The pursuit of science is also the pursuit of understanding, the refinement of human intelligence—a more serious but still grand endeavor. So understood, part of the very point of synthetic biology is *philosophy* in its original sense—love of knowledge that encompasses both physics and metaphysics. In fact, it's also philosophy in its current sense, which concerns the investigation of human systems of meaning. "The most profound and provoking question raised by the effort to build an artificial living cell," writes Regis, "was exactly the one that lurked as an unseen presence beneath all the rest: the age-old riddle, What is life?"[15]

The flip side of the value of understanding and triumphing over nature is acceptance of, even reverence toward, nature. At least to some people, the prospect synthetic biology seems to offer of still-greater human control over life is itself troubling. This is the concern that—for those who are drawn more to the human power to understand and build—is too "superficial and embarrassingly simple" to be useful.

METAPHYSICAL MISTAKES

In fact, the concern has been or could be articulated in several different ways. By and large, these formulations are neither superficial nor embarrassingly simple, but they are not all equally compelling. They depend on different philosophical commitments, and they vary in the extent to which they are legitimate bases for public policy making.

Perhaps the most straightforward way of interpreting the thought that synthetic biology amounts to "playing God" is to see it as making a fundamentally metaphysical claim, as it suggests that we humans are in some way invading divine territory. In fact, I believe three kinds of metaphysical objections might be at play in "playing god."

First, one might object that synthetic biology simply shows certain metaphysical understandings of life to be wrong. In particular, one might object that synthetic biology undermines the specialness of life by compelling us toward a reductionist view of life—by showing, that is, that life is a purely material phenomenon, a living organism no more than a complex and dynamic combination of chemicals. In the first scholarly article on the ethical issues of synthetic biology, for example, Mildred Cho and co-authors weighed the possibility that, by defining life in terms of DNA, synthetic biology reduces life to a single biological feature and therefore "may threaten the view that life is special."[16] This thought popped up again when scientists synthesized the genome of *M. mycoides*, inserted it into a *M. capricolum* cell, and ended up with a successfully reproducing line of *M. mycoides;* that achievement was heralded as debunking the idea that living things are "endowed with some sort of special power, force or property."[17] In a more recent and subtle version of the thesis, Joachim Boldt argues that "a reductionist approach to life may not be worrisome when it is only a methodological hypothesis, but if it is taken to be an ontological rather than a methodological statement, it cuts off the normative aspects of the concept of life."[18]

Boldt is right to add the qualifying "if," because the ontological conclusion is not forced on anyone. As a matter of logic, creating life in a lab cannot show that life has no special, spiritual quality. The process by which a living thing's physical body comes into being has no bearing on the existence of whatever special, spiritual qualities it possesses. A god who imbues things born in swamps and sewers with that property can do likewise if the thing takes form in a laboratory. It helps to remember that, in a sense, scientists have been creating living organisms for a long time. Every time gametes are combined in a test tube to create embryos, life has been created. Indeed, every time animals are successfully mated, life has been created. And presumably, God has been following along all the time, doing what He likes with these efforts. What changes with synthetic biology is the method, but not the basic fact, of "creation." A similar question would arise about human beings created through cloning, if that ever becomes feasible. Since a clone would be fully an individual being, possessing full autonomy and full moral powers and responsibilities, it is hard to see how that person would *lack* a soul if everyone else has one. By analogy, whatever special properties we find in microbial life generally could be found in the life of a synthesized microbe, too. In short, the fact that human beings can create a living organism does not tell us how to understand the life that the organism possesses any more than the fact that human beings can *end* a life shows us how to understand it.

What synthetic biology does show is that any alleged special, spiritual quality has no explanatory power in the laboratory, and its role in something's being alive is not testable or provable. We already knew this, really, but arguably synthetic biology shows it really well. Because of this, creating new living things in the laboratory could still bring about a change in how we think about the property of life—not by virtue of the *implications* of that accomplishment so much as by its *impact*. The development of new kinds of living things would not prove that there is no God bestowing Life on things, but it does fit well with and contribute to a story about life and the cosmos in which God has a vanishingly small and arguably insignificant role. The idea of creating living things in the laboratory would be a little like the idea that naturally occurring living things have come to be through evolution and the idea that the universe was created through a big bang and may be a random one out of an infinite many universes. These other ideas also do not prove that there is no God behind the wheel, but they do allow us to say a lot about how things have come to be as they are without appealing to the idea of God. And so the impact may be to relegate God to such a minor role that eventually we just stop referring to God altogether. Nonetheless, synthetic biology does not literally force God out of the picture. (It is an interesting quirk of the history of ideas that theists have often wanted to prove by means of pure reason that God exists, whereas atheists have often wanted to deploy empirical research to prove that there can be no God, and that neither effort can succeed, and that showing that neither effort can succeed apparently cannot succeed in discouraging either camp from continuing to try.)

This first objection to synthetic biology—or this claim about what it teaches us—makes a category mistake. Some other objections to synthetic biology accuse synthetic biology, as a field of human endeavor, of making a category mistake. The phrase "playing god," for example, suggests that humans are stepping outside their proper role in the cosmos; the category mistake is a misunderstanding and violation of the category into which humans properly go. Another way of understanding the purported category mistake is to see it as a misunderstanding and violation of the category to which living things—and life in the abstract—belong. By becoming creators of life, humans are doing something inappropriate to the items in that category. In a critique concerned primarily with the social consequences of synthetic biology, the ETC Group obliquely suggests this concern with the use of framing language such as "Original Syn?" and "The New Biomassters" (and with artwork that portrays synthetic biologists as demonic).[19] This idea is roughly the converse of the one at the start of this section: the idea is that because life is such a *very* special kind of entity, human beings dare not create it.

In a probing discussion of the ethical implications of synthetic biology, Joachim Boldt and Oliver Müller come at least very close to suggesting that synthetic biology involves a metaphysical category mistake. Boldt and Müller argue that synthetic biology has more serious ethical implications than does genetic modification because it constitutes not merely the manipulation of nature but an act of creation. "[T]his shift from 'manipulatio' to 'creatio ex existendo' is decisive because it involves a fundamental change in our way of approaching nature."[20] When we take this approach to nature, we see nature as a "blank space to be filled with whatever we wish." (Possibly, to see these distinctions between "fundamentally" different relationships to nature as implying an ontological category mistake is to read more into Boldt and Müller's language than they intend, but neither is it obviously a misinterpretation.)

The environmental philosopher Keekok Lee is more explicit. "[T]he worrying thing about modern technology in the long run may not be that it threatens life on Earth as we know it because of its polluting effects, but that it could ultimately humanize all of nature. Nature, as 'the Other,' would be eliminated." To defend against this outcome, Lee continues, "the ontological category of the natural would have to be delineated and defended against that of the artefactual."[21]

There are two kinds of category mistakes, then, that might be imputed to synthetic biology, one involving an inappropriate elevation of humans and the other an inappropriate violation of life. Strictly, if there *is* a category gap, then it should be impossible for the science to successfully breach it. Scientists could no more trespass on God's domain than they could violate the laws of physics, and if life is ontologically distinct from the physical realm, then science cannot alter *its* properties. The objection cannot be that synthetic biology achieves something humans were ordained not to achieve. Humans cannot wrongly cross a metaphysical divide; they can only wrongly *want* to. The objection must be that by pursuing synthetic biology, we humans are *representing* ourselves as God.

Very likely, to understand the moral problem in either of these ways is to believe that a very serious moral problem is at hand, since it is tantamount to believing that the proper ordering of the universe, an ordering perhaps dictated by God, is under assault. Whether very many people actually have this concern about synthetic biology is not clear, however. The reaction from the Catholic Church to JCVI's announcement that the M. mycoides genome had been synthesized and transplanted into an M. capricolum cell dismissed such worries: the announcement was praised as "a further mark of man's great intelligence, which is God's gift enabling man to better know the created world and therefore to better order it."[22] A study by the sociologist John Evans of Christians' attitudes toward human reproductive genetic technologies led him to conclude that, even when people have deep moral concerns about the relationship among God, nature, and humanity, "how humans would achieve a goal does not register to them, but rather they are focused on what the goal is....Certain goals are considered outside of the nature of the human." The goals that lie outside the nature of the human are manipulation of the nature of the human: "people thought that God had already assigned to humans...the task of healing disease, but had not assigned to humans the task of inventing themselves into new creatures with new characteristics."[23] Manipulation of bacterial life, Evans speculated, lies within the range of acceptable human goals, given the category distinctions most religions and cultures recognize among humans, animals, plants, and mere objects.

The case of chymosin is illuminating. Chymosin is an enzyme used in production of hard cheese and is found in rennet, which is produced from the stomachs of unweaned calves. (The calves need chymosin to process their mothers' milk.) The traditional way of making hard cheese is to add rennet, but an alternative approach is to produce the chymosin by means of bacteria, yeast, and fungi tricked out with cow genes. Despite all of the concern that has been raised about genetically modified plants and livestock, GM chymosin has become a fixture in the production of cheese with virtually no opposition. It was approved by the US Food and Drug Administration in 1991 and is now found in upwards of 80 percent of all hard cheese in the United States and the United Kingdom and in large percentages of cheese in some other countries.[24]

If one nonetheless holds that the alteration of microbes reflects aspirations that run afoul of metaphysical categories, still, that position does not obviously provide solid grounds for making policy. Defending that position requires appealing to and defending a rather specialized account of the ontological structure of the cosmos (and showing that the ontological structure has moral implications as well). For example, one might argue that all forms of life have been divinely created, that God gave humans the ability to create life (just as he gave them the ability to destroy it), but that he proscribed the use of that ability (just as he proscribed the ability to murder). Or, one might argue that nature is a category of things that are and should be independent of human control (as a matter of eternal fact, not merely of human moral conventions). This is the tack taken by Lee: "the primary attribute of naturally-occurring entities is an ontological one, namely, that of independence as an ontological value."[25]

I argued in Chapters 4 and 5 that public policy has a complicated stance on intrinsic values—that it should only "carve out space" within which people can live by their intrinsic moral values, but that sometimes, carving out space means providing a measure of support for a position. The policy problem posed by intrinsic values is even more complicated when the values are explicitly grounded on claims about divine purpose or ontological structure. The first point to note is that although the claims might well generate exceptionally strong moral injunctions—strong enough to generate a view that an activity should be flatly banned—public policy cannot endorse that position if by doing so it would exclude *other* moral positions that are also compatible with the basic principles of a liberal society. Second, although public policy can, in general, provide nonexclusive support for a moral position, if a position is justified expressly and particularly on religious claims or unusual metaphysical claims, then even limited policy positions may not be acceptable. Although a government could establish a park as a way of supporting citizens' beliefs about the value of nature or build a stadium partly in support of citizens' views about the value of sport, a facility built expressly in support of citizens' religious positions would probably be anathema. It seems, then, that the metaphysical case for these stances must be mirrored by or translated into broader, more secular moral considerations.

MORAL MISTAKES: THE MEANING OF LIFE

Translating the metaphysical concern into a secular moral concern can itself lead to different ways of articulating the concern. First off, one could hold that synthetic biology generates a view about the human relationship to nature that conflicts with concepts that are foundational to the practice of morality itself. In this vein, Boldt and Müller argue that by presenting organisms as machine-like artifacts, synthetic biology challenges "the connection between 'life' and 'value' [and] may in the (very) long run lead to a weakening of society's respect for higher forms of life that are usually regarded as worthy of protection."[26] Alternatively, they go on to suggest, synthetic biology might change humans' conception of human agency. With the advent of synthetic biology, humans are no longer merely manipulators of nature; they can also become creators or reinventors of nature.

The creation of nature might often be justifiable, but might also lead to overconfidence: it "might lead to an overestimation of how well we understand nature's processes and our own needs and interests and of how best to achieve them."[27]

Concerns about denigrating life and human overconfidence are secular moral analogs of metaphysical-moral concerns about violating the category of life and playing God, and some of the response to them invokes similar points. First, there is no reason to suppose that scientific investigation into how life works would force us to devalue life. The fact that an organism (be it bacterial or human) has been created in the lab does not settle what its moral value is. As Arthur Caplan wrote following the triumphal announcement of a synthetic *M. mycoides*, "The value of life is not imperiled or cheapened by coming to understand how it works."[28]

Nor need a reductionist view of bacterial life lead to a disvaluing of specifically *higher* forms of life. One study of public attitudes toward synthetic biology suggests that people are not nearly as bothered about creating and modifying single-celled organisms as they would be if synthetic biology took on the creation and modification of higher level organisms.[29] The distinctions that Evans notes are usually drawn among humans, animals, plants, and objects mean that one sort can change without others necessarily changing. People have sometimes viewed *animals* as machine-like and morally insignificant without that view having any diminishing effect on views about human life. What has been held special about human life is often not the merely biological fact of being alive, which we share with other forms of life, but an assortment of cognitive and emotional capabilities that seem to distinguish humans from animals and other living things—prominently, the capacity to have moral values and the capacity to reason. These capacities require a specialized account of some sort, above and beyond the account we would give of mere microbial life: they are emergent properties, perhaps, that microbes lack, or gifts from God, or even ways in which we partake of God's nature.[30] And since the capacity to reason gives us capacities to understand nature, to master it, and to rework it, synthetic biology might even be seen as reminding us of the value of human life. In effect, this is the other side of the claim that humans might be "playing God"; maybe we will *see* ourselves as gods. (And, in keeping with the epigram that you are what you pretend to be, maybe we will *act* more like gods. Or not!)

That we might see ourselves as gods is tantamount to Boldt and Müller's second concern, about human overconfidence. If the first point is that synthetic biology might lead us to underestimate life, the second is that it might lead us to overestimate ourselves. In particular, we might overestimate our capacity to understand and helpfully change the world. Strictly, this prospect does not seem to be an ethical problem in its own right; it does not pose the possibility of undermining the practice of morality in the same way that altering the concept of life purportedly might. The point is rather a more straightforward consequentialist one, namely, that if we get really good at this stuff, we might lose our moral moorings, use our abilities recklessly, and end up doing things that have unintended bad effects. Of course, this possibility is always there; we do not need to excel at synthetic biology in order to do things that have unintended bad effects. Our very first project might have unintended bad effects. In any event, once we see that the concern is about the consequences of misunderstanding what we are doing with synthetic biology, it is detached from any special arguments that the technology is bad in itself.

How synthetic biology might change our moral concepts might depend partly on where synthetic biology happens. If the biobricks vision really pans out and high school students working at kitchen tables are someday creating new organisms, then synthetic biology might well seem to impart a widespread human capability, and perhaps it would be likelier to have a significant effect on our view of life and humanity. But if it were restricted to the laboratory and the factory, its use monitored by regulatory authorities in some fashion, and the release of organisms into the wild forbidden or restricted, then it might be seen as a rather exceptional power—something that must be guarded and restricted and that does not broadly change the human relationship with life.

Finally, one might wonder why synthetic biology's implications for concepts generate an objection. It would not be the first time that science has challenged our views about life and our role in the cosmos. Whenever science challenges the authority of a religious text from which people derive moral guidance, the challenge has implications for moral concepts. The Copernican revolution removed humans from the center of the cosmos. The Darwinian revolution rubbed out a clear distinction between humans and other animals. In the nineteenth century, when Wöhler either presaged or launched synthetic biology by creating synthetic urea, he showed that whatever special property is possessed by living things is not causally necessary for the production of organic chemicals. It could *only* be a metaphysical property; it was not also a physical property—a kind of "vital force"—that could be isolated in the lab. But were any of these scientific developments therefore wrong? From a modern perspective, they look more like moral progress than moral decline.

PRESERVATION OF NATURE

Another way of arguing that synthetic biology raises a moral concern about the human relationship to nature is to argue that it is, in some way, damaging to nature. The environmental philosopher Christopher Preston has objected to synthetic biology along these lines. He argues that synthetic biology violates the distinction between natural and artifactual in a way that "traditional" molecular biotechnology does not. "The relevant difference," he explains, "is that traditional biotechnology has always started with the genome of an existing organism and modified it by deleting or adding genes."[31] By contrast, synthetic biology aims "to create an entirely new organism," and it thereby crosses a line that, to environmentalists, is basic and cherished: it "departs from the fundamental principle of Darwinian evolution, namely, descent through modification."

Preston's objection to synthetic biology echoes Michael Pollan's explanation (recounted in the previous chapter) for why he found GM potatoes troubling. When new varieties are created through conventional breeding, they can be seen both as products of human creativity and as an evolutionary adaptation of the plant's, but, with GM foods, the story of human creativity is a full account; the evolutionary story—the plant's perspective—drops out of the story. But Pollan's account of GM foods helps illuminate the limits of Preston's evolutionary objection to synthetic biology. Pollan did not conclude that the GM potatoes were wrong. He just didn't eat them. Synthetic organisms, like GM potatoes, lack an evolutionary story and therefore lack whatever value is unique to things that have that story, but they *merely* lack that value. They do not constitute a *threat* to that story: they do not deprive us of the value attached to that story—unless they get out of hand and become an environmental hazard.[32]

The human–nature issues that have most alarmed the public, and that have led to public policy, have concerned damage to the natural world, and especially permanent damage: when the passenger pigeon was killed off, it was gone forever. When Asian chestnut blight was introduced to North America, the American chestnut population completely collapsed. But the creation of a new kind of organism is not necessarily damaging. At least if the organism remained confined to the laboratory or factory, the natural world around us would remain unperturbed. Possibly, on the unproven assumption that the enthusiasts' hopes are well-founded, the creation of synthetic organisms will even turn out to be environmentally beneficial. In theory, synthetic biology even offers one route to a new kind of environmental restoration—species de-extinction: bringing back the passenger pigeon by synthesizing its genome in a suitable egg, transferring to American chestnuts some antifungal genes in order to confer resistance to chestnut blight.[33]

One rejoinder to this line of thought might be that, although specific applications of synthetic biology are not necessarily troubling, synthetic biology overall evinces and encourages a general view of the relationship of humans to nature that is intrinsically unattractive and could well be damaging.[34] In a penetrating paper on different views of the human relationship to nature, Bruce Jennings has suggested that we operate with a contrast between two competing discourses that might guide that relationship: on the one hand is a discourse of "altering nature to meet human demands" and on the other a discourse of "adjusting human demands to accommodate nature."[35] These discourses can be thought of as marking out two ideals (in the language of Chapter 3). The former is the ideal of building, inventing, and engineering. The latter (the "call of the wild") asks us to cherish the natural world as it is and limit the harm humans are wreaking on it—not just to keep the planet habitable for humans as long as possible, but because the planet, with its diversity of life, is valued in its own right. At least from the perspective of the latter, the ideal of building encourages us to see nature as stuff to be put to use—to be pumped out of the ground, cut down, burned, turned to waste, and disposed of as needed—and it is a human calling to gain knowledge of it, apply our capabilities to it, and, over time, develop mastery of it.

The choice between the two discourses is plainly not a straightforward either-or proposition because there is no prospect of entirely eliminating all behavior that falls under the discourse of altering nature to meet human demands. We can try to recalibrate the balance between them— to try, to the extent we can, to adjust human demands to accommodate nature. The rejoinder about synthetic biology, then, is that it fosters the ideal of adjusting nature to meet human wants and needs rather than adjusting human wants and needs to accommodate nature. It is not necessary to reduce our fuel consumption because we have a nifty technological fix (one might be led to think); we can just twiddle with these organisms to devise a brilliant new way of simultaneously producing fuel and absorbing the carbon dioxide added to the atmosphere when the fuel is burned.

If synthetic biology is really as potent as that—if it could really solve our environmental problems, or even merely be a helpful part of a larger solution—then this would be a very strange objection. It would have us, out of love of nature, disavowing something that could protect nature. The objection must be that it ultimately only makes the problem worse—somewhat in the way that adding a lane to a highway to reduce traffic congestion might ultimately encourage still heavier traffic and produce even more congestion. If this is right, then the objection needs to be spelled out: why would synthetic biology have that effect? Is there no way of using it wisely?

In fact, synthetic biology will not solve all environmental problems. There are many environmental problems that synthetic biology does not even touch—the threat to sea turtles from shrimp fishing, the draining of wetlands to build malls, the effect of light pollution on migrating birds—and those it does touch are too great to be solved by any one measure. The problems posed by the production and consumption of oil-based fuels are so vast and so serious that, even if we find new ways of producing fuels, we still need to reduce fuel consumption. In short, given the facts of the environmental crisis, even if we pursue synthetic biology, we *also* still need to alter human behavior to accommodate natural realities, and we should not suppose that the technology lets us think otherwise. There is no general choice to make between adjusting nature to human behavior and adjusting human behavior to nature.

If synthetic biology is understood as a phenomenon of the laboratory and the factory—as another way of producing things that otherwise come out of oil refineries—it is also hard to see that opting to permit applications of synthetic biology would always even reflect a *preference* for altering nature. First, insofar as it is part of a way of responding to environmental problems, we might engage in it precisely to try to alter nature less. The "green" technologies of solar power and wind power are seen as worth developing for that reason, even though, since they are cutting-edge technologies, developing them is *also* a case of developing new ways of altering nature. Second, most applications so far envisioned for synthetic biology are in the context of human activities that are not themselves expressive of the human relationship to nature. Synthetic biology is different in this regard from the genetic modification of crops and livestock. Agriculture and cuisine are human practices that, at least for many people, embody the idea that nature ought not to be changed too dramatically. The most promising applications for synthetic biology are so far in drug development and fuel production. An environmentalist will want to drive a car that does comparatively little environmental damage, but car driving is not itself an activity that reflects a connection to the earth or a conversational relationship with life in the way that agriculture and cuisine may well do. One might go into the garden—to plant or to harvest—precisely to honor one's sense of a connection to the earth, but one would just get out of the car—and walk.

SYNTHETIC BIOLOGY AND NATURE

When we consider the generic definitions of synthetic biology, the field looks to be a paradigm of human alteration of nature: what could be more significant than the application to living organisms of the principles of engineering with the goal of serving human needs? Yet when we evaluate the work on the ground—the actual applications in their social context—it is not really clear to me that it changes the terms of the game. The field touches a nerve—it raises an important, legitimate, and deep concern about the relationship between humans and nature—but when we investigate it more closely and try to articulate just how it might change that relationship, the conversation seems to spin out into inconclusive eddies. Industrial-use microbes: why not? I find I end up shrugging. Perhaps the critics have taken too seriously the enthusiasts' bombast.

Some concerns about the field are simply not well founded: synthetic biology does not show that life is nothing but a chemical process, for example, and it need not lead people either to undervalue life in general or overestimate human capacities in particular. Other concerns seem better founded, but still do not make a large moral or policy difference. Concerns grounded on metaphysical positions do not translate into policy positions very easily, for example. Concerns about its consequences for nature are mirrored by concerns about the consequences for human health and well-being that are typically less problematic bases for public policy making. And finally, as a way of changing nature, it is not obviously worse than many other things humans already do and that environmentalists regard as acceptable (if sometimes unattractive). When we consider nature under what Kate Soper calls its "lay concepts" (as described in Chapter 1), synthetic biology in its current form is not necessarily damaging to nature and does not necessarily alter the terms of the human relationship to nature. It does not necessarily change either the world in ways that deprive us of something intrinsically valuable.

To be sure, the technology could take some other form, in some new context, and end up depriving us of something we value. One way this might happen is if synthetic biology could be applied to more complex organisms or even to human beings. It might then raise the kinds of considerations discussed in the last chapter or to be discussed in the next. Also, as already suggested, the technology might end up depriving us of something that we value if it is not used wisely. The threats of bioterrorism and "bioerrorism" are worth taking seriously for the same reasons we take seriously the environmental threats posed by other kinds of industry or agriculture: not only do they pose a risk to human health and well-being, but they also may threaten naturally occurring species and ecosystems. The environmental risk raises both consequentialist concerns and concerns grounded in the intrinsic value widely given to nature. There are also very legitimate questions about the economic and social impact of synthetic biology.

A straightforward concern that synthetic organisms might damage the natural world appears to be as plausible a candidate for grounding public policy as objections about the environmental damage caused by other human activities. It requires no special defense beyond that already offered for policies to protect rare species and undeveloped lands. For most uses involving contained microorganisms, these concerns seem to run in tandem with consequentialist concerns, and, since the latter are already quite serious, the former probably do not generate any policy considerations not already generated by the latter. But this could easily change if synthesized microbes were developed expressly for environmental uses—for cleaning up oil spills or rebuilding ocean food chains, for example. Those applications might benefit humans while still posing risks to the environment—to endangered species, for example—and then the intrinsic value given to nature would be highly relevant. (And perhaps there would simultaneously be environmental benefits; there could be some difficult trade-offs to make.)

For anyone who cares morally about the human relationship to nature, the prospect of synthesizing living organisms has to be eyebrow-raising. But one must still try to assess the reaction—articulate it, explain it, and defend it. Of course, as I argued in Chapter 2, we should not expect to be able to defend our moral reactions all the way down. At the same time, as I also argued, we should expect that, at the end of the day, after we have evaluated our initial reactions, not all of them will be left standing untouched. We will have changed our minds about some. It need not be surprising or troubling, then, to find that in defending moral concerns about nature we end up shrugging off concerns about synthetic biology.

NOTES

1. Nicholas Wade, "A Decade Later, Genetic Map Yields Few New Cure," *New York Times*, June 12, 2010.
2. Edge: The Third Culture, "Engineering Biology: A Talk with Drew Endy," *Edge* 237; http://www.edge.org/documents/archive/edge237.html.
3. Ed Regis, *What Is Life?* (New York: Farrar, Straus, and Giroux, 2008), p. 6.
4. Jonathan B. Tucker and Raymond A. Zilinskas, "The Promise and Perils of Synthetic Biology," *The New Atlantis* (spring 2006), 25–45, at 25.

5. Roger Brent, "A Partnership Between Biology and Engineering," *Nature Biotechnology* 22, no. 10 (October 2004), 2011–2014.

6. Quoted in Rathenau Instituut, "Constructing Life: The World of Synthetic Biology," *The Hague, The Netherlands: Rathenau Instituut*, 2007, p. 2.

7. Rathenau Instituut, *Constructing Life*, p. 2.

8. Maureen A. O'Malley, Alexander Powell, Jonathan F. Davies, and Jane Calvert, "Knowledge-Making Distinctions in Synthetic Biology," *BioEssays* 30, no. 1 (2008), 57–65.

9. John L. Glass et al., "Essential Genes of a Minimal Bacterium," *PNAS* (January 10, 2006), 425–30; Carole Lartigue et al., "Genome Transplantation in Bacteria: Changing One Species to Another," *Science* 317 (August 3, 2007), 632–38; Daniel G. Gibson et al., "Complete Chemical Synthesis, Assembly, and Cloning of a *Mycoplasma genitalium* Genome," *Science* (February 29, 2008), 1215–20; Daniel G. Gibson et al., "Creation of a Bacterial Cell Controlled by a Chemically Synthesized Genome," *ScienceExpress* (May 20, 2010), 10.

10. S. Rasmussen, M. A. Bedau, L. Chen, D. Deamer, D. C. Krakauer, N. H. Packard, and P. F. Stadler, eds., *Protocells: Bridging Nonliving and Living Matter* (Cambridge, Mass.: MIT Press, 2009).

11. Regis, *What Is Life?*, p. 3.

12. George Church and Ed Regis, *Regenesis: How Synthetic Biology Will Reinvent Nature and Ourselves* (New York: Basic Books, 2012), 20, 68; Zunyi Yang, Daniel Hutter, Pinpin Sheng, A. Michael Sismour, and Steven A. Benner, "Artificially Expanded Genetic Information System: A New Base Pair with an Alternative Hydrogen Bonding Pattern," *Nucleic Acids Research* 34, no. 21 (December 2006), 6095–101.

13. Denise Caruso, *Synthetic Biology: An Overview and Recommendations for Anticipating and Addressing Emerging Risks* (Washington, D.C.: Center for American Progress, 2008).

14. ETC Group, *Extreme Genetic Engineering: An Introduction to Synthetic Biology* (Ottawa, Ontario: ETC Group, 2007).

15. Regis, *What Is Life?*, p. 7.

16. Mildred K. Cho, David Magnus, Arthur L. Caplan, Daniel McGee, and the Ethics of Genomics Group, "Ethical Considerations in Synthesizing a Minimal Genome," *Science* 286, no. 5447 (December 10, 1999), 2087–90.

17. Arthur Caplan, "Now Ain't That Special? The Implications of Creating the First Synthetic Bacteria," Guest Blog, hosted by *Scientific American*, May 20, 2010; http://www.scientificamerican.com/blog/post.cfm?id=now-aint-that-special-the-implicati-2010-05-20.

18. Joachim Boldt, "Creating Life: Synthetic Biology and Ethics," in *Synthetic Biology and Morality: Artificial Life and the Bounds of Nature*, ed. Gregory E. Kaebnick and Thomas H. Murray (Cambridge, Mass.: MIT Press, 2013), 35–49, at 44.

19. ETC Group, *Extreme Genetic Engineering*, 3.

20. Joachim Boldt and Oliver Müller, "Newtons of the Leaves of Grass," *Nature Biotechnology* 26 (2008), 387–89, at 388.

21. Keekok Lee, *The Natural and the Artefactual: The Implications of Deep Science and Deep Technology for Environmental Philosophy* (Oxford, U.K.: Lexington Books, 1999), 4.

22. BBC Monitoring Europe, "Vatican Dismisses Synthetic Cell's Life-Giving Dimensions, Lauds Science Research," May 25, 2010; quoted in Presidential Commission for the Study of Bioethical Issues, *New Directions: The Ethics of Synthetic Biology and Emerging Technologies* (Washington, D.C.: Presidential Commission for the Study of Bioethical Issues, 2010), 138.

23. John H. Evans, "'Teaching Humanness' Claims in Synthetic Biology and Public Policy Bioethics," in *Synthetic Biology and Morality: Artificial Life and the Bounds of Nature*, ed. Gregory E. Kaebnick and Thomas H. Murray (Cambridge, Mass.: MIT Press, 2013), 177–204, at 193 and 195.

24. GMO Compass, "Chymosin," http://www.gmo-compass.org/eng/database/enzymes/83.chymosin.html, accessed February 12, 2011.

25. Lee, *The Natural and the Artefactual*, 4.

26. Boldt and Müller, "Newtons of the Leaves of Grass," 388.

27. Ibid.

28. Caplan, "Now Ain't That Special?"

29. The Royal Academy of Engineering, *Synthetic Biology: Public Dialogue on Synthetic Biology* (London: The Royal Academy of Engineering, June 2009).

30. I owe to Mark Bedau the idea that these could be thought of as emergent properties that simpler living things do not possess.

31. Christopher J. Preston, "Synthetic Biology: Drawing a Line in Darwin's Sand," *Environmental Values* 17 (2008), 23–39. Preston revises this position, however, in "Synthetic Bacteria, Natural Processes, and Intrinsic Value," in *Synthetic Biology and Morality: Artificial Life and the Bounds of Nature*, ed. Gregory E. Kaebnick and Thomas H. Murray (Cambridge, Mass.: MIT Press, 2013), 107–28.

32. Mark Bedau has helped me clarify this stance. Bedau and Ben Larson offer a somewhat different critique of Preston's argument in "Lessons from Environmental Ethics About the Intrinsic Value of Synthetic Life," in *Synthetic Biology and Morality: Artificial Life and the Bounds of Nature*, ed. Gregory E. Kaebnick and Thomas H. Murray (Cambridge, Mass.: MIT Press, 2013), 69–88.

33. Kent H. Redford, William Adams, Georgina Mace, Rob Carlson, Steve Sanderson, and Steve Aldrich, "How Will Synthetic Biology and Conservation Shape the Future of Nature?" a framing paper prepared for a meeting between synthetic biology and conservation professionals, Wildlife Conservation Society, March 2013, http://e.wcs.org/pdf/Synthetic_Biology_and_Conservation_Framing_Paper.pdf.

34. See, for example, Bruce Jennings, "Biotechnology as Cultural Meaning: Reflections on the Moral Reception of Synthetic Biology," in *Synthetic Biology and Morality: Artificial Life and the Bounds of Nature*, ed. Gregory E. Kaebnick and Thomas H. Murray (Cambridge, Mass.: MIT Press, 2013), 149–76.

35. Bruce Jennings, "Toward an Ecological Political Economy: Accommodating Nature in a New Discourse of Public Philosophy and Policy Analysis," *Critical Policy Studies* 4, no. 1 (2010), 77–85, at 78.

CHAPTER 8

Nature in Us

Humanism and Transhumanism

There's nothing physically *wrong* with my daughters, so far as I know, but I suppose they could be still stronger and faster and so on. They're smart, but everybody could be smarter. To me, anyway, they seem sound and sensible and they're delightful to be around, but surely there are things about their personalities to adjust—if I could open up their heads, switch things around just right, and close everything up again quite safely. They are healthy, but eventually they will age; perhaps I should want to protect them not just against disease but also against decline.

Enhancements to physical form and functioning, to cognitive functioning, to mood, to moral dispositions, and to lifespan are the most high-profile issue in the contemporary debate about the human alteration of human nature. At the outer and most colorful end, the enhancement debate ventures into the "transhumanist" visions of people whose capacities and life trajectory are entirely different from those of today's humans, so that it makes sense to speak of the beings who emerge from the transition as having transcended the current species boundaries of human beings. Enhancements are not the only kind of intervention into human nature, however, and, in the near term, they may not even be the most significant. Before my second daughter was born, for example, my wife and I could have chosen to have a boy instead of another girl. Couples can also make various other choices concerning pregnancies: they can employ prenatal testing to identify certain genetic diseases or disabilities, for example, and then selectively abort unwanted fetuses. Finally, drugs and surgery can be used not only to enhance human bodies—that is, either to improve an existing capacity possessed by most normal human beings or to create a new capacity[1]—but also to "normalize" unusual bodies or even just to create unusual bodies. These interventions range from limb-lengthening for children born with achondroplasia (a form of dwarfism) to limb amputation for people who, because of a "body identity disorder," see that limb as foreign to their identity, and from pharmaceuticals to help hyperactive children sit still in class to hormone treatments that help people change their gender. The Ashley X case, in which a couple asked for both surgical and pharmaceutical interventions to stop the growth and sexual development of their severely cognitively disabled daughter and make it easier for them to care for her, is an especially dramatic case of altering a body for purposes other than enhancement.

What is the range and what are the limits of the moral attitudes that can legitimately be taken about alterations to human nature? Can it make sense to say that biomedical enhancements to my daughters are morally unappealing? This chapter defends that position, but in a complicated and limited way. Different moral stances may well be appropriate for different kinds of enhancements, I shall argue, and to the extent that one has a broad moral aversion to enhancement, the resistance may be a matter of a personal ideal rather than a public obligation.

THE CONCEPT OF HUMAN NATURE

The problem of enhancement starts with a special version of the threshold problem for concerns about nature—namely, the problem of whether the idea of "nature" or "the natural" has any real purchase. Chapter 1 introduced the problem and suggested the general outlines of a way of thinking about the concept of nature, and Chapter 5 applied that approach to the concepts of wilderness and ecological restoration. What about the concept of *human* nature?

Some commentators have argued that enhancements can be intrinsically troubling only if human nature is quite well understood. That is, there must *be* such a thing as human nature, we must have a clear account of what it is, and that account must generate reasons for not changing human nature. Arthur Caplan has succinctly articulated this claim:

> To support their position the anti-meliorists [the critics of enhancement] must state what human nature is. Despite a great deal of hand-waving about this they do not. They must also be very clear about why they see human nature as static. They

are not. And they must advance an argument about why human nature, which has evolved in response to an enormous array of random forces, accidental environmental contingencies, and stochastic genetic events, tells us anything about what is good or desirable in terms of the traits humans should possess. They cannot.[2]

I shall argue, however, that although some ways of articulating intrinsic concerns about enhancement rest on a well-developed theory of human nature, others do not. We may not actually need to be able to say just what human nature is in order to have moral concerns about changing it by means of biotechnology.

Essentialist Versus Evolutionary Views of Species

According to one long and deep philosophical tradition, to have a concept of human nature is to grasp the essence of the ontological category that (in this account) human nature is. This would be more than a mere description; it would provide a metaphysical explanation of why things in that category belong to the category. It would set out the "what it is to be" of that thing, as Aristotle's language is sometimes also translated.

To understand the essence of human nature would be to have a full theory of human nature. As classically understood, an "essence" is the concept that a particular thing embodies. The essence of a triangle, for example, is the definition of triangles that all particular triangles embody. Perhaps the essence of gold is the molecular structure that characterizes gold. An essence explains the traits that a thing has, but it is not reducible to those traits because it is unchanging and timeless. An essence has a kind of existence of its own, and, indeed, it is in a sense more real than the items that possess it (or partake of it). Further, essences are often held to relate things of different kinds to each other. An essence is unique: all of the members of a given kind share an essence, and the members of other kinds lack it. According to an ancient lineage of scholars whose work draws on Aristotle, the universe reflects God's benevolent organization—a "Great Chain of Being," so that to speak of essences is often to suggest that a kind is what it is by rational necessity and that the overall universe is also rationally ordered and necessary. We understand the order and necessity of the universe by grasping the essences that things in the universe embody.

This is a lot to take on. Fortunately, essentialism is not the only way of understanding the concept of "human nature." Essentialism models itself after an understanding of kinds in mathematics and physics, but kinds in biology are now understood along evolutionary and stridently nonessentialist lines. The evolutionary view makes no claim for the rational necessity of human nature, nor for its immutability and timelessness, nor for rationally connecting human nature to the rest of the universe. There need also be no requirement that what makes humans human is some trait that the members of other species entirely lack. Typically, looking at traits allows one to recognize species, but the traits that allow us to recognize humans as humans might all be found in some measure in other animals. And, ultimately, in an evolutionary account, what really distinguishes species is not any claim about which traits characterize the members of the species, but rather the causal story that can be told about how the species appeared on the scene and how, through reproduction, it persists. In fact, in an evolutionary account, whether a given population of animals really counts as a "species" can be allowed to remain somewhat problematic and contestable.

If the evolutionary view of species makes sense, then the term "human nature" does not demarcate the set—it does not show what counts as a human being and what does not. Instead, it functions descriptively: it tells us what the members of the set happen to be like. Of course, since evolutionary stories are also stories about how species came to be *what* they are, we expect to be able to talk knowledgeably both about traits that distinguish species from each other and about traits that species share—to describe, for example, how dogs and cats are similar and how they differ. In the evolutionary view, this is to talk about species' natures.

Claims about what dogs, cats, and other kinds of animals are like raise no special philosophical problems. And since humans are themselves animals—and *only* animals, in a Darwinian frame—then we should expect to be able to talk about human nature. Moreover, we should expect to make some headway in understanding human nature by studying our taxonomic neighbors, as Mary Midgley argues in *Beast and Man*.[3] What distinguishes human beings from other animals is typically held to be their possession of various capacities related to cognition, such as language, reasoning, tool-making, morality, and culture, but there is no need to establish that any of these capacities are possessed *only* by humans; indeed, the evidence is mounting that they are capacities or extensions of capacities that animals also possess in differing forms and degrees. At the same time, as Midgley also emphasizes, we need not restrict ourselves to biology to learn about human nature. We will have to study humans sociologically and anthropologically, as Paul Ehrlich does in arguing against adopting any unitary account of human nature and in favor of thinking that, given the significance of culture in human ways of living, there are multiple human natures.[4]

Thinking about human nature this way leads away from definitions, away from accounts that will organize the salient features of human nature under a grand theory, to straightforward lists of those salient features; but, at the same time, it makes lists unsatisfying. Perhaps the best known list is Martha Nussbaum's set of ten "central capabilities" that represent "a type of *overlapping consensus* on the part of people with otherwise very different views of human life."[5] Nussbaum includes a normal lifespan; bodily health; bodily integrity (which she explicates as being able to do with one's body as one likes); being able to imagine, think, and feel; emotionality (the capacity to love and to grieve, for example); practical reasoning; social affiliation; being able to live with concern for the natural world; play; and control over one's environment (explicated as the capacity to participate in the political and economic life of the society). Such lists often seem to be on to something; at the same time, they may seem pat and open to quibbling: Larry Arnhart offers a list of 20 natural desires "that are so deeply rooted in human nature that they will manifest themselves in some manner in every human society."[6] Arnhart includes sexuality on his list; Nussbaum subsumes that under "bodily integrity." Nussbaum includes "affiliation," Arnhart picks out "relationships" but also the more explicitly community-minded "sociality." Nussbaum includes "life" and "bodily health," but not "embodiment" per se, as Leon Kass certainly would. In short, a variety of questions arise that can look like matters of judgment: why is *this* left off? Is *that* really a general feature of human nature? Why not break that into two items? In thinking about some items, it will help to note, as Arnhart does, that the items on the list need not be true of every individual; it is enough that they are "tendencies or proclivities" that individuals possess but that are manifest on the population level.[7] It will also help to note, as both Arnhart and Nussbaum do, that the items may be instantiated very differently in different societies. Even more important is that we see all such lists as open to challenge and revision. Nussbaum stresses this point: "the list remains open-ended and humble; it can always be contested and remade."[8]

Such lists offer one way of handling, within the context of debates about human nature, the broader point made in Chapter 1 about the fuzziness of the concept of nature. Instead of a simple definition of human nature, a criterion of the sort we would expect if we looked for an essentialist understanding of human nature, we can admit that we must make do with a vaguer understanding, in which the concept is demarcated by means of an open-ended assortment of characteristics. Nussbaum's central capabilities are a starting point for a list of those characteristics. Just as we can always quibble about the list, we can also always quibble about just what counts as an enhancement. Would an alteration that reduced or eliminated a capacity—that of "relationships," say—genuinely be an "enhancement"? Or might one simply rewrite the list to exclude relationships, thereby rewriting our understanding of what is particularly important about human nature? There is no final way of resolving these debates. Indeed, we can imagine that, over the course of human history, the list of important human capabilities has already undergone some change. It might be only rather recently that control over one's environment, understood as participation in polito-economic institutions, could have made it into any widely accepted list of basic human traits.

This raises the question: why should the word "enhancement" single out *biotechnological* enhancements? Our understanding of human nature might change in part because, as Alan Buchanan has argued, recorded human history is itself, in a way, a story of human enhancement—education, written language, and the printing press are all enhancements of human function.[9] Indeed, they have changed humans biologically: our brains are different with these enhancements than they would have been without them.

In Chapter 6, I argued that we should be wary about focusing too narrowly on the genetic modification of organisms; the objection is really that agriculture in general involves ever more direct and oppressive control of nature—so that we now can think of the "industrial farm." *This* objection tells against genetic modification mostly derivatively—because it is often used to support an industrial approach to farming and because it can plausibly be seen as an especially striking example of it, insofar as genetic modification by means of biotechnological intervention is an especially effective way of altering organisms and departs from breeding's "conversational" approach to similar although more limited genetic changes. Something analogous seems to apply to the focus on biotechnology in the debate about altering human nature. Biotechnological intervention need not be seen as fundamentally different from other ways of enhancing human nature. The claim might only be that biotechnological intervention is an especially striking way of changing bodies. (There is something unusual about the prospect, isn't there? It's piqued the curiosity of movie-goers, anyway.) In principle, if not yet in fact, biotechnological interventions into human nature could have biological effects more striking than those of language and education. Also, biotechnological intervention is *into* bodies in a way that suggests top-down control of nature more strongly than do the social and environmental methods to which Buchanan compares it. The difference between them is analogous to the difference between changing the growth pattern of a plant by means of environmental alterations—giving it rich soil and planting other things around it, say—and by direct physical manipulation—pruning away unwanted branches, or injecting (hypothetical) growth-promoting chemicals under the bark, or (even more hypothetically) adding in fish genes that allow it to stay metabolically active through cold weather. (Not all of these things are generally considered troubling in agriculture, of course, and the same might hold true in human affairs.) In principle, biotechnological interventions could be the only way to subtract the capability of "affiliation" or add the capability of having a long and wonderful life *after* one has already lived a normal lifespan. Human embodiment itself has been questioned; some proponents of enhancement have outlined a future in which we get beyond interventions into bodies and make interventions that do away with bodies. Biotechnological interventions also introduce the possibility of altering human minds in a way that can introduce a disconnect between perception and reality; possibly the right pharmaceuticals could produce a feeling of intimacy where no intimacy really exists or eliminate grief in situations that seem to call for grieving, raising a question about the authenticity of experience. Finally, if a person's body has been changed by means of a biotechnological mechanism rather than through a conventional mechanism that requires as well an investment of personal effort, then, in some cases, the change can appear exogenous—the gain in athletic performance can appear to come from the pharmacist rather than the athlete.[10]

The differences between older ways of changing people and biotechnological methods are not always as sharp as critics of enhancement would like to make out, however. Sports enhancement can consist in helping the body to heal quickly, so that the athlete can train harder; treatments that used a person's own stem cells (or stem cells created from a person's skin cells) might turn out to lead to medical treatments that have a life-prolonging effect; in such cases, the biotechnological enhancement may not look quite so exogenous because the intervention seems to be working *with* as much as *in* the body. This realization simply underscores that the difference between biotechnological and other modes of enhancement is more a matter of degree than of kind. Exactly where to differentiate "enhancements" that are biotechnological interventions into bodies that make those bodies better than bodies have normally been from social and environmental changes that have mind-broadening and physique-perfecting effects (making bodies better than they have normally been) may require a certain amount of arbitrary line drawing, as discussed in Chapter 6.

Species Norms Versus Individual Differences

We would also be committed to having a fairly complete account of human nature—although a more limited theory than essentialism implies—if understanding human nature means delineating species norms for humans. We would be committed to giving an account of what features characterize any human being. (But we would not need to set out the features that distinguish human beings from creatures in other categories, as essentialism requires.)

Often, when people have discussed the role that the concept of human nature plays in moral argument, they have thought that to speak of human nature is to speak of norms and that to value human nature is to value those norms. Some have invoked human nature to argue, for example, that people can and should be sorted into two distinct sexes and that the members of those sexes have—and should conform to—typical forms of behavior, especially as concerns gender roles and sexuality. Others have dismissed the idea that there is such a thing as human nature because they see it as a convention developed precisely to support those uses.

If we subscribe to the essentialist understanding of species, then we have no option but to speak about species norms. In fact, any variation from the norms will raise awkward questions about whether the label "human" is still appropriate. But if we take the evolutionary tack, we can distinguish between claims about the species as a set—claims about what is average or normal for the species—and claims about individuals within the set. Different senses of "natural" are appropriate for claims about species and claims about individuals: sometimes, "natural" means "normal," but sometimes it refers to how individuals happen to be. Competitiveness may be typical for human beings, for example—natural in the species-typical sense—but Hannah may be innately more competitive than most—she may be "naturally" more competitive, in the second sense of the term. If we're using the first sense, then, if we attach value to nature, value is imputed to *the kind*, and deviations would be devalued. Individuals would acquire value by instantiating species norms. Under the second construal of "nature," if we value nature, then we can value individuals and diversity, and we value species norms not in themselves but simply because they help us understand individuals.

This gives us quite a lot to say in defense of human variation. Consider the view that homosexuality is unnatural and therefore wrong. Very possibly, one could argue against that view by appealing to species norms: homosexuality might turn out to be part of a *normal* distribution of human sexual nature. Analogously, no one would say that people who are uncommonly athletic lie outside the range of normal human behavior and that their athletic behavior is therefore inappropriate. Whether sexual attraction to the same sex is natural in the sense of being "normal" is, of course, both an empirical question and a question about where one draws lines through continuous statistical curves to demarcate "the norm." But if we are interested in nature in the sense of innate, individual variability, we can also defend homosexuality more directly: we can say that this is how some people find themselves in the world and that they should be who they are. I suspect many will share this intuition. Similarly, consider ambiguous genitalia and other intersex conditions. In the past, doctors have often taken immediate action to disambiguate these conditions, surgically altering children so that they would look more plainly male or female. That sort of action was driven at least in part by the first construal of nature. But if we are thinking along the lines of the second construal, we would likely say that there is some value in leaving ambiguous genitalia just as they are, even though they are certainly atypical.

Valuing variability will not make us blind to kinds and norms, and there will be situations in which we still need to talk about kinds. In arguing against enhancement in sports, for example, one would want to offer some assertions about the range of normal human functioning—the levels of erythropoietin one can typically expect to find in a person's blood, for example, or the sorts of cases in which a person could be said to have a testosterone deficiency (and the levels of testosterone that therapy should aim to achieve). But this is an indirect way of bringing norms into consideration. The starting point is nature in the second sense—that in which "nature" refers to what we find in the world, in all its individual diversity, rather than to species norms. The norms may be explicitly recognized as somewhat arbitrary cut-offs. And it is what we find in the world that is the locus of value: the point of sports is partly that they celebrate the variety of natural—innate—human gifts found among athletes, including some extraordinary departures from norms.[11]

Along these same lines, might we also find value in *dis*ability—in physical attributes that depart from the norm in the direction opposite that of professional athletes? A common theme among those who think about human disability is that we find a way of accepting and valuing "the anomalous, even the pathological, and [that] we must do so if we are to proceed with our varied lives in a satisfactory and satisfying manner."[12] This is not necessarily to say that human disability or difference is *desirable*—as if we ought to work to *achieve* it by creating disabilities.[13] It is to say only that one can value the stance of *accepting* these differences, if they have arisen "by nature."

Here, too, a recognition of norms comes into consideration indirectly because it is only against the background of the normal bell curve that the anomalous is identifiable. Of course, calls to "accept" differences must be made and handled very carefully. Norms can also be used to set people apart from the moral community. As Nussbaum points out, to note that some people lack, by nature, certain typical human capacities—that they are "disabled"—can give cover to stigmatization and discrimination. "The use of terms suggesting the inevitability and 'naturalness' of such impairments masks a refusal to spend enough money to change things on a large scale for people with impairments."[14] This may at times be true. But to show that a moral term is covertly used to justify bad behavior does not reveal a problem with the moral term itself; one can justify a kind of cruelty by emphasizing the importance of honesty, yet that does not reveal a problem with honesty. And, as Nussbaum herself notes, whether a variation in human capacity amounts to a "disability" is often a function of human decisions about the way society and its institutions are designed. To acknowledge this fact is to decouple questions about whether an impairment is acquired "by nature" and whether (for example) a building ought to be redesigned to make it more accessible to more people.

Nussbaum's underlying concern in arguing against justifying disability by appeal to nature is that we not justify unjust ways of distributing resources. Justice, as she understands it, requires that we ensure that all human beings, to the extent possible, possess a full set of basic human capabilities, and this can require a greater commitment for people born with certain kinds of differences—not a pat acceptance that nature stood in the way. It is not clear, however, that this goal prevents us from simultaneously finding some value in leaving natural human variation alone, even when it amounts to disability. If our moral values are all merely facets of a single general conception of the good, rather than a heterogeneous and incommensurable lot, then, whenever we seem to have to choose between accepting human difference and promoting justice, one or the other must win out without any loss of value. Deciding that justice requires producing normal human capacity could not leave a sense that eliminating human difference was unfortunate—the value of accepting human variation would have to disappear in whatever case was at hand. If we think values are heterogeneous and incommensurable, however, one could admit a residual moral loss even while reliably preferring to bring people up to normal human capacity. Understanding the decision this way helps make sense of cases in which one finds some value in leaving a body alone: one way of making the value of accepting human variation disappear is to deny that it is ever there at all, but this runs against the intuitions many have about disability and difference, perhaps particularly when we consider interventions that merely normalize appearance and do not directly affect human capacity in any way. (Nussbaum herself may be gesturing at thoughts along these lines: she holds that if very severe disabilities could be permanently removed by means of genetic engineering, then they should be, but that conditions which, although disabling, leave open a real chance of achieving the crucial human capabilities, might not be.[15])

The tension between accepting human variation and promoting normal human capacities has to do with how moral *values* stack up against each other, but an uncertainty about the very concept of human nature underlies it. "Human nature" can refer both to how individual human capacities are acquired and to general claims about human capacities. Human bodies and faces tend to look so and so, and that is a fact of nature, but there is also a surprising degree of variation, and that, too, is a fact of nature. However, both in rejecting the essentialist understanding of human nature and in allocating only a limited role to assertions about human species norms, we shift the focus from broad claims about what human beings are like to a recognition of diversity, complexity, and individual variation. And to do so is to give up pretensions to a commanding knowledge of what human beings in general are really like. We can say a little about human nature in general, but we are really more interested in individual human nature.

Of course, identifying individual human nature is a complicated business. Individual human nature is not purely a matter of biological inheritance, but also of culture and creativity. We are who we are partly because we are simply built that way but also partly because of environmental influences (a causal relationship that, experienced from inside it, can be indistinguishable from biological inheritance) and partly because we have allowed ourselves, or perhaps tried very hard, to be that way. The degree to which a given trait can be said to be caused purely by biological influences (by raw nature, as it were), by culture, and by individual decisions will vary from trait to trait, but we can plausibly say that human beings are, in a very significant way, fundamentally self-creating beings, both in the sense that they live in cultures that form their natures and in the sense that the possession of human capabilities makes possible the construction of one's being. In effect, it is part of human nature that we develop our own natures and influence the natures of people around us. As a result, the idea from Chapter 5 that "natural" is to be explicated historically, by weighing the relative causal contributions of nature and humanity, is significantly complicated when we consider human nature rather than wildlife and wildernesses. It's still harder, when we consider human nature, to sort those contributions out.

THE VALUE OF HUMAN NATURE

I hope to have shown so far that the "antimeliorists" need not meet Caplan's challenge to "state what human nature is" head on. A "great deal of hand-waving" will suffice, if the hand-waving consists in showing that we can talk sensibly about the nature of human beings without exactly having a "theory of human nature," much less one that shows human nature to be static. But what about Caplan's requirement for an argument showing why human nature ought to be left alone?

Like claims about what human nature is, arguments about the moral significance of altering human nature can take different forms. In the typology I offer here of these arguments, I want to move in two contrasting directions at once. On the one hand, I will try to shore up the "antimeliorist" position to the extent I can. However, my strategy will be to set aside the kinds of arguments that genuinely seek to mount arguments for keeping human nature, in general, static and to argue instead only that the decision not to change human bodies can be a legitimate moral stance to take. In effect, then, I may be offering an addendum to Caplan—an important and interesting one, I hope—rather than opposition. The problems with some antimeliorist positions are often rooted, as Caplan points out, in the claims they presuppose about what human nature is—or about what an account of human nature is. Different positions have different implications for what one must know about human nature.

Human Nature as an Inviolable Ontological Category

Previous chapters have considered various ways in which the value of nature is sometimes claimed to be grounded in ontological distinctions— that things whose existence cannot be credited to intentionality are metaphysically or ontologically distinct from the artifactual, that species are fixed categories of reality, and that life is a property that humans may not "synthesize." Similarly, human nature might be considered ontologically distinct. Something is ontologically distinct when it is distinct not merely superficially—not merely on the basis of observable features—but in terms, instead, of its very *being*. Mind, for example, is sometimes thought to exist on its own right, rather than as a feature of the physical world; if so, it is ontologically distinct. Classes, too, are sometimes thought to exist in their own right, rather than merely as assemblages of individual things. This is the view of human nature that goes along with talk of the essence of human nature. The essence—the "what it is to be" of that thing—defines the class to which individual human beings belong.

If we hold that ontological categories are not merely figures in the fabric of the cosmos but that they also generate limitations and obligations concerning what humans *may do* in the cosmos, then we have the strongest sort of argument for why we should not alter human nature. It is here that we find the argument, "X is against nature, and therefore wrong"—the argument considered at the start of Chapter 3, and perhaps the sort of argument that Caplan asks critics of enhancement to produce. Language like "going against nature" or "violating nature" implies this kind of position; things are not being filed in their right places. Such a serious moral error might well make any other moral consideration otiose.

It may be that objections to atypical sexual behavior are often supposed to be based on ontological claims. One might think that human nature is divinely ordained and that it is a feature of human nature that people are divided into two distinct sexes—"male and female created He them"—and that human behavior that does not conform to these basic lines is divinely *hated* and therefore wrong. But this is not the only way of talking about the value of human nature.

Human Nature as a Source of Moral Guidance

A closely related and also very strong claim about the connection between human nature and moral values is that the concept of human nature is a source of moral guidance. This position tries to accept only the last half of the previous position: it holds that human nature generates moral limitations and obligations, but without making controversial stipulations about God's purposes or Being's categories. But it, too, commits one to a strong understanding of human nature.

Of course, everyone can agree that *some* knowledge of human nature is important for moral judgments: values lead to specific moral positions only in light of premises concerning relevant facts. But to say that human nature is the basis for morality is to go a step farther and hold that human nature provides not only factual premises but value premises as well. Leon Kass is often thought to exemplify this way of thinking about the moral relevance of human nature and about human enhancement. Certainly, there are glimmers in Kass's writings of this approach. He sometimes speaks of human nature as a kind of touchstone or guiding light in thinking about biotechnology. *Beyond Therapy*: Biotechnology and the Pursuit of Human Happiness, a report on enhancement produced by the President's Council on Bioethics, for which Kass was chair and intellectual leader, asserts that, "only if there is a *human* 'givenness,' or a given humanness, that is also good and worth respecting, ... will the 'given' serve as a *positive* guide for choosing what to alter and what to leave alone."[16] Also, it is striking that, although the Council evaluated enhancements case by case, it reached skeptical conclusions about any change that is not a paradigm case of treating a disease; the method is case by case, but the agenda general.[17] Finally, there is an undercurrent of essentialism in Kass's writings. Kass emphasizes the limits of science and empiricism and the room—and need—for alternative ways of apprehending human life. "Our current evolutionary orthodoxy," he notes, "has, in fact, little to say about the true origin of life or about ultimate causes, not only of life but of all major biological novelty. It cannot account for the emergence of higher organisms."[18] We need to turn, Kass tells us, to "unorthodox biologists," and in particular to Aristotle, "who emphasized questions of being over becoming, form over matter, purposiveness over moving parts, and wholes over parts; for whom the soul was not an ethereal spirit or a ghost-in-the-machine but an immanent and embodied principle of all vital activity; and for whom science was a refined and ever-deepening reflection on the natures and causes of the beings manifest to us in ordinary experience."[19]

It is hard to read such passages without concluding that Kass thinks, at some level, that the cosmos is rationally ordered, that humans—highest of the higher organisms—have their proper place in the overall order, and that understanding their nature is not merely a matter of collecting observations about what humans are like but is also a matter of gaining special insight into larger mysteries.[20] These grander ambitions for how the concept can be deployed in moral thinking suggest a commitment to a much stronger theory of human nature than Kass ever attempts to provide.

Kass's views are complicated, however, for he also explicitly *denies* that he sees human nature as a source of moral guidance.[21] Moreover, his method is not what one would expect of someone who saw human nature as a source of moral guidance: someone who thinks human nature provides moral guidance would probably first set out an account of human nature and then apply it to domains of human behavior. But Kass's method is typically to start by considering questions about the *meaning* of human behavior and how biotechnology can change it. In a chapter about the creation of human embryos in the laboratory, the philosophical discussion begins with a section subtitled "The Meaning of the Question," and Kass explains that his "orientation" is "that before deciding what to do, one should try to understand the implications of doing or not doing."[22] Kass then connects these, not to an account of human nature, which would offer various claims about what humans *are*, but to the "idea of humanness," which is a question about how we think about ourselves—a topic for poetry as much as for science.

This method seems to commit Kass only to a limited theory of human nature. He is making claims about what is species-typical for humans, but the claims do not amount to a complete account of what is human and what falls outside the category. Moreover, the claims he offers are about such basic features of human life—sexual procreation, growing old and passing away—that they encompass not only all humans, but all animals. Kass's approach, under this second interpretation, is best rebutted not by challenging his claims about human nature but by challenging his claims about meaning.

On the other hand, claims about the meaning of human behavior are not the strongest way of making a general case against enhancement. If one turns to an account of the meaning of human behavior, then it is possible to follow the case-by-case method that the Council suggests but end up with case-specific rather than general conclusions. (This is the route followed by Thomas Murray, and it is described briefly later.) Drawing a clear but general moral line between enhancement and therapy—objecting to enhancement while accepting therapy—seems to need a full, strong theory of human nature. To establish that line, we would need to show that "enhancement" refers to interventions that move individuals outside the category of human nature and "therapy" to interventions that preserve or return individuals to human nature, but we then need to be able to explain both what the category is (referring not just to individuals in it but to the defining characteristics of the category itself) and why it must not be violated. This is to make human nature a source of moral guidance (Kass's disavowal to the contrary), and it is, as Caplan and many others have noted, a very challenging undertaking.

Human Nature as a Condition of Morality

Another way of thinking about the moral relevance of human nature is to see it as a necessary condition of morality. That is, moral obligations are "grounded" in something else, but their content cannot be specified except by recourse to some understanding of human nature. Human rights, for example, presuppose some understanding of what humans need, claims about human equality presuppose some idea of what humans are typically capable of, and claims about human autonomy presuppose some understanding of human agency.

Francis Fukuyama's argument against human enhancement rests on this kind of approach. To make the argument, however, Fukuyama is forced to develop a fairly elaborate account of human nature—for it is only if the necessity relationship between morality and an account of human nature is quite tight that changing human nature raises problems for morality.

Fukuyama claims that human nature "is the sum of the behavior and characteristics that are typical of the human species, arising from genetic rather than environmental factors."[23] This is an attempt to avoid a traditional form of essentialism; we are to think of human nature not as something *definable*, but as an overall set of traits. Fukuyama therefore does not try to offer a complete list of these traits, and, in fact, the set would have to be somewhat indeterminate, if only because—as noted earlier—any attempt to specify "fundamental facts" tends to be indeterminate. Further, the set will consist of ranges of traits rather than of precisely specified traits. Indeed, because traits are actually a function of environmental as well as genetic factors, an account of traits "arising from genetic factors" will be unstable; "normal human height," for example, can change over the generations due to changes in diet. Nonetheless, out of this deliberately rough understanding of the range of traits possible, given the human genome, emerges what is distinctively human, which Fukuyama calls "the human essence" or "Factor X." This is not itself a trait, but an emergent property that depends on the entirety of human traits:

> If what gives us dignity and a moral status higher than that of other living creatures is related to the fact that we are complex wholes rather than the sum of simple parts, then it is clear that there is no simple answer to the question, What is Factor X? That is, Factor X cannot be reduced to the possession of moral choice, or reason, or language, or sociability, or sentience, or emotions, or consciousness, or any other quality that has been put forth as a ground for human dignity. It is all of these qualities coming together in a human whole that make up Factor X.[24]

The problem with enhancement technologies, for Fukuyama, is that if we shift human nature beyond the pale of the traits that our genes make possible, then we will disrupt "the ground for human dignity" and therefore for human rights. Given his understanding of "the human essence" as emergent from the overall set of human traits, Fukuyama maintains a broad opposition to enhancement. "What is it we want to protect from any future advances in biotechnology? The answer is, we want to protect the full range of our complex, evolved natures against attempts at self-modification."[25] In other words, it is not only language and rationality, but the entire set of human behavioral and physical characteristics that concern Fukuyama. Fukuyama's opposition is also stringent: the apparent implication is that even relatively small changes—giving humans greater height or strength, for example—might be threatening.

There is something in Fukuyama's position that is interesting and plausible, but there is also much about it that is slippery. Morality is undoubtedly pegged to some features of human nature; to speak of autonomy is to assume that human beings have the capacity to set their own goals and follow them, working to overcome desires that get in the way, for example. But that capacity is part of a thin understanding of human nature. Fukuyama's claims about the qualities that come together to make up Factor X amount to a much richer understanding. Is the richer account compelling? Since Fukuyama does not describe the key qualities, the problem cannot be that he gets human nature *wrong*. But he lays out some parameters for how they come together to make up Factor X, and the problem is that these parameters cannot get us to a point where, if we maintain a detailed account of human nature, we can ever be confident we have human nature right. Yet, without a detailed account, the opposition to enhancement loses power.

The relevant traits are supposed to be genetically determined human species norms. The idea is that we can identify the traits we must watch (even if the list is open-ended), fix their appropriate ranges, and sort out the genetic contribution to them. One problem is that sorting out the genetic versus the environmental contribution to traits has proven very difficult—difficult enough that, as Ehrlich argues, we can speak ultimately only of human natures, not of human nature. Another problem is with the idea of fixing the ranges well enough to identify what falls into and what outside the human category. This easily leads to some perplexing results, as Nicholas Agar has shown.[26] It may imply, for example, that Shaquille O'Neal, whose height is certainly anomalous, is not quite human. Fukuyama is aware of this danger, and he takes pains to stress that traits vary greatly and that gene–environment interactions can shift the entire range of traits over time. He allows that "There are doubtless some mutant female kangaroos born without pouches"—kangaroos, in spite of the fact that having pouches is part of "kangarooness."[27] A universal need not literally be universal; "it needs rather to have a single, distinct median or modal point, and a relatively small standard deviation."

Perhaps a latitudinarian approach to variation keeps us from going astray on what human nature is, but it then tends to make rigorous opposition to enhancement difficult to sustain. If we allow that Shaquille O'Neal is a man, then we might also be able to say that a physically rather significantly enhanced human is not, as the title of Fukuyama's book proposes, "*post*-human." Enhancement that does not bump a person beyond the range of normality might be unobjectionable, or at any rate enhancement that shifts someone outside the range of normality might not *always* undermine the basis for human dignity and human rights. Enhancement would seem to pose a problem only when it occurs often enough and dramatically enough to pull apart the statistical curves that describe normal ranges of human traits. It is broad social trends that we would really have to be concerned about, not individuals.

A third problem is with the very idea of identifying the key traits to watch—the traits whose ranges determine human nature. Fukuyama is flirting with essentialism, as his language suggests, without quite wanting to go there: although an indeterminate list of traits that human beings possess does not amount to a definition of what it is to be human, Fukuyama nonetheless wants to say that human beings constitute a distinct and fixed category that can be given a unique definition. An element of mysticism seems to creep in at this point: there is something ontologically special, only we cannot say what it is, and our inability to say what it is means we should be *especially* cautious about proposals to change it. But, insofar as we see the position as sneaking in essentialism, it looks hard to sustain.

But perhaps there could be a more resolutely nonessentialist version of the argument that human nature is a condition of morality. Paul Lauritzen argues that if biotechnology can significantly change human capabilities and life trajectories but is not available to most people, then it risks undermining our common sense of humanity, which could undermine the capacity for human sympathy. [28] The starting point for this thought is that human identity is bound up with human biology, such that "a new biology might give rise to a new psychology." A new psychology would lead, in turn, to a new ethics. In particular, worries Lauritzen, it would challenge our conception of human rights. "The most persuasive account of human rights," he writes, "is framed in relation to the notion of a stable human nature." The fear, then, "is that biotechnology will change the species-typical characteristics shared by all humans. If that happens, and if rights are tied to a conception of human nature that is in turn rooted in a biological reality, then biotechnology threatens the very basis of human morality as we know it."

In Lauritzen's view, then, it is critical to human morality that there is a stable human nature and that humans all recognize that there is a stable human morality. But "a stable human nature" does not imply *unique* human nature. Lauritzen is not concerned that we can show what is in and what is outside the category. His point seems to be only that we must have some ability to describe important human characteristics and considerable confidence that people of different races, ethnicities, sexes, and nationalities share them in roughly the same measures. We might start in the way Nussbaum does, by developing lists of key human capacities, while acknowledging that the lists are always open-ended and contestable. To do so is to speak of human norms, but it is not to make the norm itself the locus of value. In short, Lauritzen is not committed to anything more than an ongoing exploration of human nature. But it is also not clear that Lauritzen is committed to as stringent a line against enhancement as Fukuyama seems to want to defend. It is only very significant and population-level changes, unequally available to the population, that his argument tells against.

The Relationship Between Humans and Nature

Another way of arguing for the moral significance of human nature is to argue that a certain kind of relationship to it is morally significant. This is, in one respect, a simpler way of trying to explain why human nature is important. The previous three approaches all try to establish that an understanding of human nature is *necessary to explain moral values*: human nature is a necessary condition of important moral concepts or is itself a source of moral guidance, maybe even an ontologically special source of guidance. The idea in this fourth approach is merely to say that, wherever moral values come from, the relationship humans have to human nature is a topic that is morally important. Instead of arguing that human nature generates moral constraints on enhancement, that is, those who take this approach argue that moral views about human nature generate moral constraints on enhancement. The complexities enter the picture when the values are explicated.

Michael Sandel and Jürgen Habermas exemplify this approach: Sandel argues that a certain relationship to human nature is both valued in itself and vital for various other valued things, and Habermas argues that a certain relationship to human nature is vital for equal membership in the moral community.

Sandel's argument for worrying about enhancement is broad-ranging, and, in places, he seems to develop arguments that follow consequentialist lines. The point he emphasizes most heavily, though, is that certain ways of using enhancement lead to an imbalance in two sorts of relationships to human nature—an accepting relationship, in which we see nature as a gift, and a perfectionist relationship, in which we strive to improve it. The ideal is to hold these in tension with each other, but enhancement pushes us away from the first and toward the second. Widespread use of enhancement would "represent the one-sided triumph of willfulness over giftedness, of dominion over reverence, of molding over beholding."[29]

Sandel goes on to say why losing "the ethic of giftedness" would be unfortunate, but these final observations may work more to elaborate on the misfortune than to explain it. Losing the ethic of giftedness would undermine "three key features of our moral landscape—humility, responsibility, and solidarity." This claim could be understood as a consequentialist point—if we lose these key constraints on our behavior, many people will end up worse off—or it might be understood as pointing out conceptual implications—if we lose these aspects of the "moral landscape," we could not but feel that as a huge loss. Sandel plainly hopes, though, that many of his readers will feel the loss of giftedness *itself* already as a loss. It is partly to show the import of losing giftedness itself that he tries to show how it is bound up in sports and in parenthood, such that if we lose the ethic of giftedness, then sports and parenthood will be diminished—"the drive to banish contingency and to master the mystery of birth diminishes the designing parent and corrupts parenting as a social practice governed by norms of unconditional love."[30] Sandel's argument is not limited to sports and parenthood, however; he intends these discussions to exemplify a larger point about giftedness.

For the moment, the important point is that Sandel can speak of the human relationship to bodily nature without making any overarching claim about human nature other than that the traits people have are a function of the bodies they have and that, traditionally, people have acquired their bodies and therefore their traits through contingent processes rather than through design. The point of giftedness is that we do not know exactly what to expect in human nature, and we should foster an "openness to the unbidden" (a phrase he draws from William May, who served with Sandel on the President's Council on Bioethics). But such claims fall well shy of a theory of human nature.

Habermas's case against enhancement begins with the thought that living in communities and engaging each other as equals is possible because we all share a "prior ethical self-understanding"—an understanding of who we are that makes it possible for us to see ourselves as "ethically free and morally equal beings."[31] Critical to this self-understanding is that we are embodied beings—animals, not angels—and that our bodies are *our own* in the sense that we do not acquire them from others in the community; they are products of fate or nature rather than of design. In short, a certain way of being related to one's own body is a condition of being one's own person—of having autonomy, of having unique worth, of being a member of equal standing in the moral community. We must be able to assume that "we act and judge *in propria persona*—that it is our own voice speaking and no other."[32]

Habermas worries that this assumption is at risk if a child knows that it has been genetically enhanced by its parents, for then the parents' goals are present directly in her body, as it were—not merely through the familiar processes of child rearing and socialization, which also impose others' goals on the child but which the child can, in principle, reject. Habermas supposes that these goals will not be present in children's bodies in the same way. Of course, children might accept the parents' goals as their own, and, if they do, they will not feel deprived of their own voice. But the possibility that the child's and the parents' goals will not harmonize needs protecting; genetically enhancing one's children "jeopardizes a precondition for the moral self-understanding of autonomous actors."[33] Thus, parents should approach parenthood with an "expectation of the unexpected" (a phrase Habermas draws from Hannah Arendt).[34]

The idea that parents should expect the unexpected strikes the same chord as Sandel's borrowed line that we should be open to the unbidden, and that similarity seems to me to be the key point in understanding Habermas. Habermas's argument could be understood as positing a claim about human nature—namely, that traits are not acquired from others' designs—and then showing that this claim is a condition for autonomy and community. This would put Habermas's position in the same category as Fukuyama's—as positing that human nature is a condition of morality. But I read Habermas as working alongside Sandel, not Fukuyama: the argument starts with the thought that we *value* the fact that our bodies are not derived from others' designs, that they are arrived at with a heavy mixture of contingency, and it proceeds to the claim that this "ethical self-understanding" also contributes to other aspects of our moral lives.

Also like Sandel, Habermas is advancing claims about human nature that are modest and defensible. He is not making claims about human beings' essential nature, nor about a normal human range of traits. There is no thought that we have thoroughly catalogued the traits that make up human nature, much less that we have come up with a *definition* of human nature that sets out a criterion for those traits. Indeed, neither Sandel nor Habermas identifies any *particular* desirable human traits that humans generally ought to have; neither is concerned with norms. It is the *relationship* to human nature as found—to individual differences—that they are concerned about. For each, it is enough to say that individual human beings come into the world with their own natures. They argue that for us to assert (too much) control over others' natures is troublesome. Nor does either imply that human nature is fixed. Human nature might indeed change; Sandel and Habermas assert only that there is value in allowing the change to be contingent.

The complexity of the genes' contribution to actual human life may qualify Habermas's and Sandel's concerns about asserting control over how children turn out. Certainly, it complicates them. Parents' success at using genetic technologies to *make* their children turn out one way rather than another is likely to vary greatly, depending on what traits they have in mind for their children, and it may well be that most of the traits parents would want to produce, and in particular most of the most interesting traits, lie beyond genetic control. Success at controlling a trait might not be necessary for intervening in it to raise a concern, however. Parental control over a child's nature might still be a problem if an intervention falls short of controlling the child's nature but leaves a lasting reminder for the child—on the child—of what the parents wanted the child to be (although more needs to be said about whether lasting bodily reminders of parents' plans would affect the child's sense of its autonomy). Sandel's worry that the child is not seen as a gift depends on the parents' attitudes, which (Sandel supposes) depend in part on parents' capacity to carry out their own plans; but, in specific cases, parents might entirely fail to regard a child as a gift even though they have little or no ability to exchange the child's given traits for ones they would prefer. Plainly, then, both Habermas's and Sandel's concerns are matters of degree. (Sandel is explicit on this score, since he frames his concern as a point about the balance between two competing attitudes that stand in tension with each other.) Worries about parental control of children would grow as parents are able to affect how their children turn out.

If concerns about genetic interventions are explained in terms of parents' attitudes and children's self-understanding, then, plainly, too, there is no sharp line demarcating genetic from environmental interventions. To the degree that an environmental change leaves an ineliminable reminder of the parents' own intentions for the child (consider the behavioral conditioning that is imagined in *Brave New World*), then it ought to generate Habermas's and Sandel's concerns every bit as much as would happen if the effect were accomplished through genetic intervention. The genes are not special repositories of value, to echo a point introduced in Chapter 6. The guiding thought is rather that the relationship in which we stand to our human nature(s) and to the natures of our children—the degree to which we seek to alter or seek to accept (to pick up on language developed in Chapter 7)—is a matter of human value.

Human Nature and Human Flourishing

Sandel and Habermas argue that the human relationship to nature is intrinsically important but understand that claim in a more modest way than their critics sometimes suppose. They mean only to express the value of accepting human bodies as they are, not to advance grand assertions about the normative significance of fixed ontological categories or general species norms. Also, both are making somewhat limited claims about the value of letting bodies be—Habermas about the undesirability of parental intervention in children's bodies and Sandel about striking the right balance between intervention in bodies and acceptance of bodies.

If claims about the value of human nature are appropriately limited, then they can creep into moral thought through a side door, without necessarily even being recognized as claims about the value of human nature. Consider some who argue that the relationship between humans and nature is intrinsically important in particular contexts or that there are particular aspects of human nature that are intrinsically important.

One narrower, more cautious kind of approach is marked out by Thomas Murray, who suggests that we think of human nature as providing "the contours of the given" and then consider the implications of changing those contours for specific social practices. The social import of some practices—their meaning—depends on having certain complex relationships to the human given and can be undermined if it is altered by means of biotechnological shortcuts. On the topic of enhancement in the context of sports and parent–child relationships, for example, Murray and Kass are not far apart: enhancement is at odds with the meaning of sports, Murray writes, because "what we look for in athletes is a combination of *natural talents* and the *virtuous perfection* of those talents."[35] Athletic competition can be conceived of along different lines, Murray observes, but then the meaning of the practice is different—so different that those competitions seem distinguishable from "sports." They are about maximum performance instead of natural talents honed through hard work. Somewhat similarly, enhancement of children is at odds with the values that shape the parent–child relationship: it is important that parents accept their children "as they are, with their appetites and enthusiasms, fears and aspirations, however that personal reality might diverge from our idealized image of the child we dreamt of having."[36] Murray frames his objections to enhancement as claims about human flourishing, on grounds that the social practices he examines contribute to the human good, and he concludes that enhancement is not in general a bad thing; in some cases, what is plainly enhancement would even be desirable. If surgeons could safely take pills that steadied their hands or allowed them to remain alert through long surgeries, they should do it.[37] Again, it is explicitly an understanding of the social practice from which we take our cue. Still, the underlying point is that, in certain social practices, accepting human bodies as they are is intrinsically valuable. Claims about human flourishing and the value of human nature tend to run together at this point.

Murray, too, is not committed to an overall theory of human nature. His claim is not that human nature in general is valuable, but that, in some contexts, we have reason to value human nature as we find it. If sports are for us an opportunity to celebrate natural talent, for example, then we will be concerned about aspects of human nature relevant to sports—strength in weightlifting, for example, the blood's oxygen-carrying capacity for bicycling, and ability to slow one's heart rate in archery. At the same time that some enhancements are barred from sports, others are incorporated; bicycles and tennis rackets are sometimes said to be mechanical enhancements of a sort. The bicycling enthusiast need not have thought that *all* human enhancement is wrong, but only that, given the way the sport of bicycling is constituted, *certain* human enhancements are undesirable.

Another version of this limited approach to thinking about human enhancement would be to make general—non-context-dependent—claims about specific aspects of human nature, again without being committed to a complete account of human nature. The philosophical movement known as "transhumanism" helps bring this point out. As the very name suggests, transhumanism tacitly rests on some understanding of human nature. Rather than valuing human nature, however, transhumanists see it as a condition that we not only may but should strive to transcend. Generally, by transhumanists' lights, we should rid ourselves of the animal portion of our nature. We should be free of the constraints of our bodies, free perhaps of bodies altogether, much smarter than we are, and much longer lived (ideally immortal). If we were largely cut loose from our bodies, we might also have different views about sexuality and music and the value of social affiliation.[38] Other aspects of human nature—especially pleasure and the capacity to set goals and deliberate about how best to pursue them—would be retained (and refined).[39] But whereas transhumanists have some ideas about how we should get better, they need not have a complete account either of what we are or of the species we are to become. Exactly what we would turn out to value, once we reached our new state, might be entirely impossible for us to say in our present limited state.

Conversely, one whom we might think of as a "mere humanist" might value an assortment of things about being human—items from Nussbaum's and Arnhart's lists—without having a complete account of the kind of being we should remain. If we set aside the hints in some of Kass's writings that some grander, essentialist understanding of human nature underpins the opposition to enhancement, then this more limited approach might be his method. (Conversely, to the extent that Kass sees human nature as a special ontological category, then perhaps he should be dubbed a "*transcendental* humanist.") This more limited understanding is also consonant with Lauritzen's, Sandel's, and Habermas's conclusions, although they base their conclusions on somewhat more specialized arguments.

The mere humanist can allow that there is no account that conceptually ties together all of the items on the list, and she can acknowledge that the list is open-ended and contestable; hence, there is no grand theory of human nature in play. The mere humanist also does not have a grander argument for why those items appear on the list (any more than the transhumanist has an argument for why pleasure is to be sought). Consider "emotions," which Nussbaum puts in the fifth place on her list of basic human capabilities: "Being able to have attachments to things and people outside ourselves; to love those who love and care for us, to grieve at their absence; in general, to love, to grieve, to experience longing, gratitude, and justified anger."[40] Having emotions is a feature of our animality, and perhaps emotions are a feature of our animal nature that we might, in some bizarre future transhumanist world, be able to diminish and reject. But it does seem to be a feature of human life that a humanist would value.

Statements about the value of humanity tend to blend at this point with statements about "human flourishing." Nussbaum holds that the ten basic human capacities are the minimal conditions for a life with human dignity. Jonathan Glover makes a similar point in a marvelous set of essays on the breadth of parents' freedom to choose the kind of children they wish to have. Glover seems at one point to set concerns about the intrinsic value of human nature to one side:

> In the early days of the debate on genetic enhancement, some of the objections raised (such as that it would be "un-natural") were based mainly on emotional revulsion ("the yuk factor"). Some people still have this kind of revulsion. But one result of twenty years' discussion is that these responses have been questioned and largely put aside. Now the serious debate is in the spirit of the harm principle and reflects concern for people. The impact of genetic enhancement on human flourishing, on the kinds of lives people will lead, is central.[41]

In the closing section of his book, however, Glover contemplates that parents' choices may need some sort of restraint, and he considers several possible bases for these restraints—to prevent social inequalities, to keep parents from falling into self-defeating competitions, to protect the child's right to an open future. "And, perhaps most fundamentally, the limits may be needed to protect parts of human nature needed either for the containment of our dark side *or else in a more positive way for the good life, parts of our nature that it would be tragic to lose*."[42]

Glover has reason to say that losing valuable parts of our nature raises a concern about *harm to human flourishing* rather than the *value of human nature*: articulating the concern in that way seems less likely to lead to

blanket statements in the way that claims about human nature are sometimes thought to do. Perhaps, too, it encourages a more considered moral
position, since we recognize the necessity of weighing different ways of
flourishing. (What's really objectionable about "the yuck factor" is its seem-
ing thoughtlessness.) But to identify a basic human capacity that we deeply
value and *want to preserve* in human lives—the capacity to have emotions,
to participate in communities, to have values, to deliberate morally, to love
music, to share humor—is to say something more than that human flourishing is a good thing and harm to human flourishing is our guide. It is to
make particular and richer claims about human flourishing that are also
claims about human nature as it has existed up until now. We may not be
objecting to enhancement across the board, by any means, but we are certainly objecting to altering certain aspects of human nature.

Claims about the value of human nature can also be seen as structurally similar to environmentalists' claims about the value of the natural
world outside humans. Why resist human enhancement? Potentially,
for a variety of possible reasons: in particular cases, because enhancement conflicts with the value of a practice, or undercuts the authenticity of experience, or seems likely to be self-defeating or futile. But often,
maybe, only because we value nature—here, nature as found in oneself—
and therefore aim for a relationship toward it that accepts it—a preservationist stance toward *human* nature. It is tempting to try to provide an
argument, as Caplan asks us to do, but in fact, at times, there might be
no argument we can provide beyond pointing again to the value we find
in nature. Concern for nature can be a brute feature of our moral lives.

LETTING BODIES BE: HUMAN NATURE
AND MORAL IDEALS

Some of the positions just canvassed are challenging to sustain. They make
claims about human nature and about its normative force that cannot be
supported. Some others have less taxing commitments. They depend neither on a full theory of human nature nor on a theory of morality that
supposes claims about human nature are pivotal to morality. They propose,
instead, that we start from inside our values: from claims about giftedness,
for example, understanding giftedness merely as articulating a point about
a human relationship to nature that is valued in itself, and without further
explanation, rather than as a claim involving an actual giver of some sort.
Or we might begin, as perhaps Kass, as Murray, and as transhumanists and
Glover do, from basic claims about the human good (understanding those,

too, as calling attention to things that are valued in themselves and without further explanation).

None of the more defensible positions gives conclusive reasons for prohibiting enhancement across the board—for regarding them as violating publicly enforceable moral obligations—although the limits to their ambitions are not always clear. Allen Buchanan, describing himself as "anti-anti-enhancement," argues that Kass, Fukuyama, Habermas, and Sandel appear to be trying to provide *conclusive* reasons against enhancement because they marshall arguments against enhancement, say little about arguments for enhancement, and often sound strident.[43] But there's another reason they might concentrate on arguments against enhancement and sound strident when they do: they might be trying to shore up a position that they think is in danger of being overwhelmed. Rather than shutting down the other side, in other words, they may simply be trying to avoid getting shut down themselves.

One of the great problems with the debate about human enhancement is that it so easily looks like a debate about which of two contrasting positions will silence the other. This would make sense if the debate were about whether human enhancement is impermissible, as Buchanan interprets Kass and others to be saying—or about whether it is obligatory, as John Harris thinks.[44] The complex account of value outlined in Chapter 3 was meant to block out another way of thinking about moral concerns about the human relationship to nature, however; the idea there was that those moral concerns may mostly fall not into the realm of obligation and permissibility—of enforceable standards that govern human interactions and can be modeled on the conceptual framework of a contract—but into the realm of ideals by which people orient their identities and plan their lives—standards that an individual may feel obligated to follow and may encourage others to follow but which he or she does not regard as flatly obligatory for others.

In fact, it would be possible to hold that some forms of enhancement are impermissible, some are required, and some (simply) conflict with moral ideals to which individuals may be deeply committed. The human enhancements that might be prohibited, at least partly on grounds that they conflict with important intrinsic moral values, are those that would undermine "parts of our nature that it would be tragic to lose." (Alternatively, because intrinsic and consequentialist considerations collapse into each other when we are discussing core aspects of human nature, we might describe opposition as being grounded in the harm principle, as Glover proposes, but bearing in mind that our conception of harm rests on a rich conception of the human good, one that is explicated in much richer terms than "pleasure" or "happiness.") One set of potentially tragic changes to human nature are those that Lauritzen contemplates: enhancements that manage to undermine human solidarity. Imagine changes that led to a new speciation event among humans, as Lee Silver once proposed: enhancement technologies cause some portion of the population to, in effect, split off into a separate population, reproductively and maybe communally walled off from those who either decide against enhancement technologies or (in Silver's imagined future) lack access to them.[45] The separated group might also have their own institutions for education, governance, entertainment, and so on. Or imagine that the transhumanist vision of uploading minds into machines and dispensing with human bodies could be achieved. Significantly extended human lifespan might also tend to undermine human solidarity, if the extended and unextended humans come to believe that they have fundamentally different sets of interests.

One important caveat about Lauritzen's concerns is that enhancements would have to occur at a species level, not merely to a few individuals here and there, in order to undermine human solidarity. This means that individual enhancements themselves might not always be worth prohibiting; however, actions that promoted species-level changes—policy decisions that might drive individual enhancements en masse, for example—might be objectionable. A more significant caveat is that the kinds of enhancements that could undermine core parts of human nature are still the stuff of science fiction; they are not yet possible. Dramatic change to human nature may never be likely, given the complexity of genes and traits, and might be impossible to try in morally acceptable human experiments.[46] And, anyway, given the desirability of basic human goods, it seems unlikely that, even if it were technically possible, enough people would adopt such changes that they would amount to species-level changes. Yet less dramatic interventions—improving human cognition by 40 IQ points, extending average human lifespan by 40 years, or making a 4-second 40-yard dash a fairly common accomplishment seem unlikely to undermine human solidarity.

A special category of traits whose loss would be tragic are those aspects of human nature that are necessary for good moral judgment. If we assume, as Chapter 2 argued, that moral deliberation depends on proper functioning of emotional nature, not just on an ability to reason well, then we can imagine enhancements that undermine moral functioning. Perhaps some enhancements to cognition would subtly change moral feeling (making the person more intelligent but less reasonable). One can also imagine that greater personal assertiveness, which some would undoubtedly view as an enhancement, might correlate with limited instincts of empathy and solidarity. Similarly, some transhumanists have envisioned human beings who lack the urge many humans have to socialize.[47] Enhancements that damaged moral functioning might not be intrinsically desirable to enough people that they would lead to species-level changes. Even if done only on an individual level, however, they might be deeply objectionable and warrant out-and-out prohibition.

The prospect of damaging moral feeling leads to a more difficult question. There are other features of human nature that are less likely to lead to bad social consequences—that at least would not undermine morality—but whose loss might be tragic, even in individuals. Perhaps these include love, musical expression, and a sense of humor. Suppose that C. P. Snow's image of "two cultures" also describes alternative kinds of human minds—a scientific and technical mind and a humanistic and artistic mind—and that, unfortunately, these dispositions turn out to exclude each other within the human brain, just as Snow feared they were excluding each other in human society. The scientific and technical sort is a kind of *Star Trek* Spock—logical, knowledgeable, and articulate, but incapable of processing human emotions. On the off chance that it were scientifically possible to create a human mind that did not particularly suffer but also did not partake deeply (or at all?) of ordinary human thrills, could this kind of enhancement represent a loss of intrinsic human goods so serious as to be impermissible? Hopefully, the scenario will never actually present itself: either the human mind will not be modifiable like that or a mind modified like that will not be attractive to anybody.

Even if some enhancements warrant a ban, some other enhancements might warrant support of some sort. If vaccinations are essentially enhancements of the immune system, then they are an obvious candidate. Or what about injected nano-bots that function like powerful vaccinations? Another candidate for an enhancement that could, in some distant future, plausibly be made mandatory would be behavioral alteration that improved moral deliberation and strength of will, such as by enhancing the human capacities for impulse control, sympathy, altruism, or moral imagination.[48] In a fractured and violent world where powerful weapons are easy to come by, constraining the seemingly natural human tendency to violence might become essential. (Note that none of the moral enhancements listed here would relieve one of the need to think about what one is doing; none of them would *cause* a person to do the right thing.) Perhaps there are also settings in which particular human functions could be made mandatory, along the lines of Murray's example of enhanced muscle control in the surgical theater. The US military has already put us on this path by sometimes requiring Air Force pilots to take modafinil to prolong wakefulness.

Given this back and forth, there is no one general rule governing the overall moral acceptability of enhancements. In fact, the range of cases just discussed probably establishes that there is no one general conclusion to be reached only about the *intrinsic* moral desirability or undesirability of enhancements—that the variation in overall moral acceptability is not just because desirable consequences sometimes override the intrinsic undesirability of enhancement. Enhancement may not be *generally* intrinsically undesirable. Some features of human nature are bad and warrant improving, and some features of human nature that are not bad are still sometimes worth improving. Our relationship to our own human nature can nonetheless be a matter of intrinsic moral concern, at least in the complex and modest sense that one may hold that accepting human bodies as they are (as well as human behaviors and everything else that goes along with having a human body), as if they were a gift, is a moral ideal one strives to find a way of living by. One way of articulating the complexity and modesty is to point out that there is a contrasting ideal of self-improvement and that the ideal of accepting bodies as they are ought somehow to coexist with it.

Can we balance these contrasting considerations? It is tempting to aim for simplifying things and say that one must either endorse improvement and reject acceptance or endorse acceptance and reject improvement. But think of the attitude one may take toward an actual gift—a box of different kinds of cookies from a grandmother. I could plausibly decide to dispose of some of the cookies that are bad for me or that I dislike (some have nuts, which we will imagine I am allergic to, and some have pieces of candied fruit, which I simply loathe), and I might trade some away for other, better cookies (I found someone who will take candied fruit in exchange for ginger snaps, which I can eat in quantity), and yet I could still believe that I should be grateful to my grandmother for the cookies, and I could in fact be grateful, and I could decide to alter the box of cookies to a limited degree (I will keep a few of the cookies with candied fruit because they are traditional in my family and in hopes that I can come to like them, and I will keep all of the squishy, brandied brown things, even though I am not terribly fond of them). I now have an enhanced collection of cookies, but I have simultaneously sought to uphold the value I put in accepting the gift as it is.

The case is similar, I believe, with the more closely analogous case of preserving natural environments. It is possible to hold simultaneously that wild nature ought to be preserved and that we will cut some trees down to build a fire and clear some land for a garden. Thomas Hill's example of a morally unattractive stance toward nature (considered in Chapter 3) depicts a man who cuts down all of the trees on his property and paves the whole area, but what if the neighbor carefully preserves everything except a patch of a particular flowering plant? Let us say the plant gives him hay-fever, or he fears it will become invasive, or it attracts pests that will dam-age some of the other plants, or he simply really dislikes that plant. I think that if the man ripped out this plant, we could still credit him with acting on a preservationist ideal toward the nature on his land. There are differ-ent values held in tension, with none of them functioning as trump cards that always cancel out the others and no neat way of articulating how they should be weighed against each other.

These contrasting standards are analogous to the competing discourses discussed in Chapter 7. In discussions of human enhancement, Erik Parens is the foremost advocate of this line of thought. Different views about enhancement technologies rest on different "ethical frameworks," suggests Parens. "As one side emphasizes our obligation to remember that life is a gift and that we need to learn to let things be, the other emphasizes our obliga-tion to transform that gift and to exhibit our creativity."[49] Most people lean toward one or the other of these stances toward enhancement, but most people also understand and adopt both stances to at least some degree. Some enhancements are more likely to arouse a sense that the human body should be left unaltered. (Parens proposes a pill to create a feeling of inti-macy between two people whose actual interactions with each other do not show intimacy.) Others are likelier to arouse a sense that heavily altering one's body is entirely appropriate (Parens considers sex change operations here). And about many kinds of enhancements, we will be genuinely per-plexed and ambivalent, drawn in some measure toward both views.

If there is a difference between preservationist instincts about the envi-ronment and about human nature, it is that, when we turn to human nature, the preservationist instinct arguably includes a meliorist instinct within it. If human beings are, to a significant extent, self-creating beings, then the instinct of enhancement can itself be understood as part of human nature and engaging in enhancement as a way of honoring human nature. We can be ambivalent about altering the environment because there are differ-ent values at stake and because we may have difficulty deciding whether the state of affairs we have in front of us should count as "natural" or not. When we think about altering human nature, perhaps we can be even less sure that a human causal contribution moves us away from a "natural" state. Human nature as we find it and human nature as we create it are not just hard to distinguish factually, but to some degree at least, lead concep-tually into each other.

Some may see this difference as making a complete hash of any attempt to make sense of the ideal of accepting bodies as they are. I tend to see it, instead, as compounding the complexity of achieving a balance between the competing ideals, giving yet more reason to be tolerant of different views about altering human nature, and being wary of buttressing any given view in public policy. The enhancements that might be impermissible and the enhancements that might be obligatory are mostly very significant enhancements and are mostly not yet live options for anybody. The more realistic possibilities for the near future are comparatively minor enhancements—to form, as in cosmetic surgery; to physical function, as in steroid use; and to some aspects of behavior, as with caffeine and methylphenidate (Ritalin) to enhance focus, modafinil to prolong wakefulness, and alcohol, cigarettes, and certain kinds of antidepressants to enhance mood. By and large, with enhancements like these, impermissibility and obligatoriness are not in question. This is a domain for personal moral choice, a domain that includes ideals that drive individuals' choices but do not generate social obligations.

In this domain, the challenge for public policy is to figure out how to "carve out" space for those who want to live by the ideal of letting bodies be, without inappropriately imposing the value on everybody. Often, probably, this can be accomplished simply by permitting individuals to make their own choices about how they will enhance their bodies. There will, of course, be several familiar complications. One of these will be presented by cases in which parents seek enhancements for their children. Parents are often granted wide leeway to make decisions on behalf of their children, at least when their children are quite young. But what about a case, described by Alicia Ouellette, in which a father arranges blepharoplasty for an adopted Asian daughter, causing her "sleepy" eyes to open wider and look more Caucasian?[50] Ouellette argues that the daughter may, later in life, come to wish that the epicanthic folds in her eyes had been preserved, as she might come to regard them as an important physical connection to her ethnic identity. Similarly, the daughter might come to feel simply that her own bodily nature was worth preserving. Such cases suggest, Ouellette argues, that parental authority to make body-modifying decisions for their children should be constrained. There will be a spectrum of kinds of body modification, however, ranging from blepharoplasty to vaccination (where the alteration has clear medical benefits) and circumcision (which may have no medical benefits but is entangled, in a very different way from blepharoplasty, with questions about social group cohesiveness, the importance of fitting in with a social group, and religious freedom), and, within this range, some kinds of body modification will be untroubling or even mandatory.

Another kind of complication will concern group or state decisions that constrain individual decision making. Many critics of enhancement have considered the possibility that if deciding whether to use enhancements is regarded as a matter of individual choice, then social pressures may, over time, make it increasingly difficult to choose against enhancements. If the majority of a state's citizens end up opting for enhancement, however, it is not clear why the state should take measures to protect the way of life of those who would prefer to opt against them, if protecting their way of life means something more than preserving individual choice among the options that the society makes available. Nor is it quite clear just what the state *could* do. If the social pressures were severe (as the critics suppose), then carving out a space might amount to creating a parallel, non-enhancement-endorsing society, which is more than could be expected.

One way the state might be able to carve out space for those who want to live by the ideal of letting bodies be is to allow the formation of private associations that cleave to that ideal, extending the principle of individual choice to the group level. (In a way, the state would be permitting the formation of non-enhancement-endorsing societies within society.) This is what happens when a sports-governing body such as the International Association of Athletics Federation (IAAF), which oversees track and field, forbids certain kinds of enhancements. The IAAF turns to the World Anti-Doping Agency (WADA) to determine what will be considered suitable for "the spirit of sport," and WADA periodically draws up lists of unacceptable enhancements.[51] In effect, WADA is working through the difficulties in the concept of nature—the gray areas caused by the impossibility of demarcating "natural" through a single simple criterion—by considering a spectrum of examples, case by case, much as Nussbaum gives us a list of the "central capabilities" of human beings and much as the organizations that enforce particular understandings of "organic" agriculture work through an assortment of cases and draw up lists of the agricultural practices that will not be considered organic. (The list-making strategy for developing policy was also discussed in Chapter 6.) Of course, it would also be permissible to set up *pro*-enhancement sports governing bodies, and, indeed, that has happened in weight-lifting.

Still, the question remains of what the state can and should do, whether it may adopt policies that steer individuals toward enhancement or attempt in any way to slow down the development of enhancement technologies. One measure the state could take, of course, is (simply) to promote careful public deliberation about enhancements, to ensure that individuals are considering the implications of their choices and making their choices wisely. This seems to have been the chief goal of the President's Council on Bioethics. "[T]he concerns we have raised here emerge from a sense that tremendous new powers to serve certain familiar and often well-intentioned desires may blind us to the larger meaning of our ideals," wrote the Council, at the very end of its magnum opus on enhancement.[52] The broad societal goal, concluded the Council, should be to benefit from biotechnology without losing "our founding ideals." The Council's own goal in drafting a report on enhancement was to "spark and inform a public debate, so that however the nation proceeds, it will do so with its eyes wide open." Promoting such public discussion would promote wiser choices both for individuals and for society. Promoting wiser choice is itself a way of giving air to different ideals, but it can also allow those who lean away from enhancement to articulate their stance as well as possible and win others over as much as possible.

At the end of the debate, a liberal society could permissibly opt to engage in what Allen Buchanan calls "the enhancement enterprise." A society would embark on that program, Buchanan says, when it not only assures that members of the society are free to develop and use enhancement technologies but also provides public resources to support the development of enhancement technologies and public deliberation about their wise use.[53] Financial support for the development of enhancement technologies may well have the effect of promoting enhancement technologies as a viable moral option and may draw support away from the ideal of letting bodies be, but this outcome seems to be acceptable, if enough people are inclined in that direction. Conversely, a liberal society might also opt against providing financial support for the development of enhancement technologies and might even take measures to actively support a human nature-preserving ideal. As noted in Chapters 4 and 5, there is an element of majoritarianism in deciding how much support to provide to concerns about nature. Government support for environmental preservation, even to the point of enacting freedom-constricting legislation such as the Endangered Species Act, is warranted partly because moral concern for the protection of environmental nature has a lot of public support. Similarly, if, after a careful public debate in which respectful attention is given to both sides, the public tends to opt away from enhancement or opts only toward certain enhancements or only toward comparatively modest enhancements, then public policy could reasonably back away from the full "enhancement enterprise." In particular, it could decide against providing financial support for enhancement. That might have to come from the private sector.

A DELIBERATIVE ENTERPRISE

Some of the theoretical positions I have staked out in this book are out of the mainstream, maybe even radical, at least for bioethics. The account of the concept of nature and of the nature of values is drawn from work in environmental ethics and from long traditions of thought in Western philosophy that lie behind that work, but they are not widely shared in bioethics, which generally aims for a more orderly and objective view of morality. The notion of a moral ideal, which gives reason for thinking that moral goals about the human relationship to nature might not translate easily into public expectations, and the contrasting idea that a liberal society may legitimately take positive actions to carve out space for its citizens' values—which gives reason for cautiously translating private moral standards into public positions—may also be somewhat unusual.

Yet the practical positions I have taken are, in many ways, not very radical. Also, they are not very specific. I have not shown when to protect a wilderness, where to put a wildlife sanctuary, when to support a restoration effort, or when to opt for development, nor have I presented a method that could reliably churn out those answers. Nor have I marked out a clear path forward on human enhancement. I have tried, rather, to show how the arguments must go, and I have really tried to explain why the arguments are frustrating and difficult, as much as I have tried to clean them up. Indeed, I have defended and perhaps even compounded the complexities: I hope to have given reason to be cautious about any pat formulae or principles for sorting them out, and I hope to have given reason to think that appeals to nature are a legitimate part of these debates, but also that they are not a decisive part. I have argued that the idea of wanting to preserve, protect, or remain content with natural states of affairs is not always an irrational or mystical position, as critics often suppose. It can be an ordinary although not central moral view people hold, and it can even legimately influence the formation of public policy in a liberal society. For the time being, then, the way forward is not the enhancement enterprise, but the societal endeavor to articulate, expound, and examine our deeply felt positions on our growing power to alter the world.

NOTES

1. This definition is similar to that offered by Allen Buchanan, *Beyond Humanity?* (New York: Oxford University Press, 2011), 23.
2. Arthur Caplan, "Good, Better, or Best?" in *Human Enhancement*, ed. Julian Savulescu and Nick Bostrom (New York: Oxford University Press, 2009), 201.
3. Mary Midgley, *Beast and Man: The Roots of Human Nature* (London and New York: Routledge, 1979).
4. Paul Ehrlich, *Human Natures: Genes, Cultures, and the Human Prospect* (New York: Penguin, 2000).
5. Martha Nussbaum, *Women and Human Development: The Capabilities Approach* (Cambridge, U.K.: Cambridge University Press, 2000), 76.

6. Larry Arnhart, *Darwinian Natural Right: The Biological Ethics of Human Nature* (Albany, N.Y.: State University of New York Press, 1998), 29.

7. Arnhart, *Darwinian Natural Right*, 30.

8. Nussbaum, *Women and Human Development*, 77.

9. Buchanan, *Beyond Humanity?*, 23ff.

10. President's Council on Bioethics, *Beyond Therapy: Biotechnology and the Pursuit of Happiness* (Washington, D.C.: President's Council on Bioethics, 2003), 143–44.

11. Thomas H. Murray, "Enhancement," in *The Oxford Handbook of Bioethics*, ed. Bonnie Steinbock (New York: Oxford University Press, 2007), 491–515.

12. Eva Kittay expresses this thought by saying that we "normalize the anomalous." Eva Kittay, "Thoughts on the Desire for Normality," in *Surgically Shaping Children: Technology, Ethics, and the Pursuit of Normality*, ed. E. Parens (Baltimore, Md.: Johns Hopkins University Press, 2006), 90–110, at 100.

13. Adrienne Asch, "Appearance-Altering Surgery, Children's Sense of Self, and Parental Love," in *Surgically Shaping Children: Technology, Ethics, and the Pursuit of Normality*, ed. E. Parens (Baltimore, Md.: Johns Hopkins University Press, 2006), 227–52, at 248.

14. Martha Nussbaum, *Frontiers of Justice: Disability, Nationality, Species Membership* (Cambridge, Mass.: Belknap Press, 2006), 188.

15. Ibid., 193.

16. President's Council on Bioethics, *Beyond Therapy*, 289.

17. Ibid., 22.

18. Leon R. Kass, *Life, Liberty, and the Defense of Dignity: The Challenge for Bioethics* (San Francisco, Cal.: Encounter Books, 2002), 288.

19. Ibid., 294.

20. Ibid., 296; Kass emphasizes the importance of mysteries here.

21. Kass, *Life, Liberty, and the Defense of Dignity*, 296.

22. Ibid., 85.

23. Francis Fukuyama, *Our Posthuman Future: Consequences of the Biotechnology Revolution* (New York: Farrar, Straus and Giroux, 2002), 130.

24. Ibid., 171.

25. Ibid., 172.

26. Nicholas Agar, *Liberal Eugenics: In Defence of Human Enhancement* (Oxford, U.K.: Blackwell Publishing, 2004), 96.

27. Francis Fukuyama, *Our Posthuman Future*, 135.

28. Paul Lauritzen, "Stem Cells, Biotechnology, and Human Rights: Implications for a Posthuman Future," *Hastings Center Report* 35, no. 2 (2005), 25–33, at 28.

29. Michael Sandel, *The Case Against Perfection: Ethics in the Age of Genetic Engineering* (Cambridge, Mass.: The Belknap Press, 2007), 85.

30. Ibid., 82–83.

31. Jurgen Habermas, *The Future of Human Nature* (Cambridge, U.K.: Polity Press, in association with Blackwell Publishing, 2003), 38–41.

32. Ibid., 57.

33. Ibid., 63.

34. Ibid., 58.

35. Murray, "Enhancement," 513.

36. Ibid., 508.

37. Ibid., 503.

38. Asher Seidel, *Immortal Passage: Philosophical Speculations on Posthuman Evolution* (Lanham, Md.: Rowman & Littlefield Publishers, Inc., 2010).

39. Nicholas Agar, "Whereto Transhumanism? The Literature Reaches a Critical Mass," *Hastings Center Report* 37, no. 4 (2007), 12–17.

40. Nussbaum, *Frontiers of Justice*, 79.

41. Jonathan Glover, *Choosing Children: Genes, Disability, and Design* (New York: Oxford University Press, 2006), 76.

42. Ibid., 103, emphasis added.

43. Buchanan, *Beyond Humanity?*, 59

44. John Harris, "Enhancements Are a Moral Obligation," in *Human Enhancement*, ed. Julian Savulescu and Nick Bostrom (Oxford University Press, 2009), 131–54.

45. Lee Silver, *Remaking Eden: How Genetic Engineering and Cloning Will Transform the American Family* (New York: HarperCollins, 2007).

46. Norman Daniels, "Can Anyone Really Be Talking About Ethically Modifying Human Nature?" in *Human Enhancement*, ed. Julian Savulescu and Nick Bostrom (Oxford University Press, 2009), 25–42.

47. Seidel, *Immortal Passage*.

48. Buchanan, *Beyond Humanity?*, 56.

49. Erik Parens, "Toward a More Fruitful Debate About Enhancement," in *Human Enhancement*, ed. Julian Savulescu and Nick Bostrom (Oxford University Press, 2009), 181–97, at 189.

50. Alicia Ouellette, "Eyes Wide Open: Surgery to Westernize the Eyes of an Asian Child," *Hastings Center Report* 39, no. 1 (2009), 15–18.

51. World Anti-Doping Agency, "The World Anti-Doping Code; The 2013 Prohibited List"; available at http://www.wada-ama.org/Documents/World_Anti-Doping_Program/WADP-Prohibited-list/2013/WADA-Prohibited-List-2013-EN.pdf.

52. President's Council on Bioethics, *Beyond Therapy*, 309–10.

53. Buchanan, *Beyond Humanity?*, 16.

INDEX

achondroplasia, 157
adult, definition of, 9
aesthetic value, 23, 38, 58, 121
Agar, Nicholas, 172
Air Force, 184
alfalfa, 112
All Creatures Great and Small, 125
American Prospect, The, 29
Amyris Biotechnologies, 139
antidepressants, 187
AquaBounty Technologies, 113
Arendt, Hannah, 176
Aristotle, 26, 158, 169. *See also under*
    moral theory
Arnhart, Larry, 39, 160, 179
artemisinin, 139
artifacts, 1, 6, 8, 42, 49–50, 93, 95–96,
    98–99, 146, 167
Ashley X, 46, 60–61, 157
assisted suicide, 75
authenticity, 121, 162, 181
autonomy, 32–33, 172, 175

Bacillus thuringiensis, 113
Beauchamp, Tom, 30
benefit, definition of, 9
benefit of future generations, 5
Bentham, Jeremy, 30
Berry, Wendell, 101, 106
*Beyond Therapy: Biotechnology and the
    Pursuit of Happiness*, 168
biobricks, 137, 148
bioethics, 4, 9, 22, 25, 81, 84
biotechnology
    agricultural, 4, 109–111,
        122–23, 137
    and concept of enhancement, 158,
        161–62

and moral arguments about
    enhancement, 76, 168–69, 171,
    173, 189
and synthetic biology, 137, 149
bioterrorism, 140, 152
Blackburn, Simon
    on moral sentiments, 25, 27
    on nature, 28
    on the "staircase of practical and
        emotional ascent," 36–37, 38, 57
    on truth and relativism in moral
        judgments, 32, 34, 35
blepharoplasty, 187
body identity disorder, 157
Boldt, Joachim, 142, 144, 146–47
Bovenkerk, Bernice, 109
Brave New World, 177
Buchanan, Alan, 161, 182, 189
Bunning, Jim, senator of Kentucky, 62

Callicott, J. Baird, 24, 28, 31, 37
"call of the wild," 49–50, 57, 150
Caplan, Arthur, 147, 157–58, 166–68,
    181
Catholic Church, 145
central dogma, 115
Certified Naturally Grown, 128
Charles, Prince of Wales, 109, 124
chestnut, American, 89, 124, 149–50
chicken, 109–110, 115
Childress, James, 30
Cho, Mildred, 142
chymosin, 145
circumcision, 187
climate change. *See* global warming
cloning
    animal, 110
    human reproductive, 28–29, 43, 142

CPSIA information can be obtained
at www.ICGtesting.com
Printed in the USA
BVHW042102210819
556456BV00008B/54/P